Taekwondo Spirit & Practice

Author's Previous Books:
Tae Kwon Do: The Korean Martial Arts, Harper Collins Publishers
Advancing in Tae Kwon Do, (Harper Collins), United States
    Taekwondo Association
Moo Duk Kwan; The Korean Art of Self Defense, Ohara Publications
Advanced Moo Duk Kwan, Ohara Publications
Numerous instructional videos on self-defense

Taekwondo Spirit & Practice

Beyond Self-Defense

Grandmaster Richard Chun
with
Richard LaMarita

YMAA Publication Center
Boston, Mass. USA

YMAA Publication Center
4354 Washington Street
Roslindale, Massachusetts, 02131
1-800-669-8892 • www.ymaa.com • ymaa@aol.com

ISBN:1-886969-22-1

10 9 8 7 6 5 4 3 2 1

Publisher's Cataloging in Publication
(Prepared by Quality Books Inc.)

Chun, Richard.
    Taekwondo spirit & practice : beyond self-defense /
Grandmaster Richard Chun with Richard LaMarita.
    —1st ed.
    p. cm.
    LCCN: 2002108594
    ISBN: 1-886969-22-1

    1. Tae kwon do. I. Title. II. Title: Taekwondo
spirit and practice

GV1114.9.C48 2002   796.815'3
                                           QBI33-597

Printed in Canada

Contents

Preface

I am telling my story at the age of 67. I have been involved in the practice and teaching of Taekwondo for more than half a century. When I think of that, I am awestruck. It is unbelievable that a choice I made so innocently at the age of 11 has played such a major role in shaping who I am and the road I would take in this journey called life.

Truly, life is a mystery. How does one find his path? Was my meeting with the martial arts accidental or predestined? Were my choices ones that came from the heart or from the mind? The story I am about to tell will share my experiences in the martial arts and how they have shaped both my life and myself as a human being. It is clear to me now that any other life would not have been more right for me.

When I first began my practice of Taekwondo, it was mainly a means of physical development. I enjoyed the discipline and hard work that the training required. I was committed to it and, as a result, developed good work ethics. I became strong and healthy. These qualities remained with me and benefited me throughout my entire life. Even now, discipline and hard work are the tools I use to achieve my goals. Having this foundation, I am never disappointed in my endeavors.

Gradually, I began to sense a deeper meaning in my training. The mental attributes that a young martial artist develops came into the foreground. Slowly and naturally, a sense of inner strength and a peaceful state of mind blossomed within me. This manifested itself in a reassuring fearlessness towards life. I felt that I could overcome any obstacles that stood in my way. These mental attributes complimented continuing physical development. It was exciting to see that my study of the martial arts was expanding and deepening, and that I was expanding and deepening as well.

As I grew into manhood and became a Grandmaster of Taekwondo, I realized that ultimately the martial arts were a spiritual discipline and practice. The physical and mental development continued, but added to this was the profound understanding that being a martial artist meant becoming a whole person. I saw that everything in my life was touched by my martial arts experience; its influence was pervasive. As I grew aware of this, I began to feel invincible, yet humble. I finally understood the truth behind the famous warrior maxim that states, "A man who has attained mastery of an art reveals it in his every action." To be a true master in the martial arts is to be a master of one's own life and destiny,

As a master, it became my mission to teach and communicate to young martial artists the completeness of the path they were choosing. I never wanted any single part of their training to overshadow the whole, because each part contributes equally to create a stronger and more complete entity.

To this end, all my life and work has been dedicated. As a constant reminder of this process, nothing gives me greater pleasure than conferring black belts to my students. When a new student comes to me, they are in essence asking for my guidance in their journey. When a student earns his black belt, I know that I have passed on a deep tradition. I have fulfilled my responsibility as a friend, teacher and mentor.

Earning a black belt in my school means much more than just passing a test on forms, sparring, and breaking. A black belt signifies not only physical excellence, but mental wisdom as well. My students must also take a written exam to see how much knowledge of the tradition and philosophy they have absorbed. I like to see that they have learned the true purpose of becoming a martial artist. Only after I read their answers do I know if they have truly achieved black belt status. Only then will I pass the black belt to them.

Throughout my forty-five years of teaching, I have rewarded over several thousand black belts to students. Nevertheless, each time I am moved by the tradition. I pass the black belt to the student in the presence of their family, friends and other students and assistant instructors with whom they have trained. The new black belts lined up on the gym floor in their doboks. I approach each individual and say his or her name for all to hear, holding a new black belt in my hand. We bow to each other and I tie the black belt around their waist. Then we bow again to each other and I congratulate them. This simple gesture symbolizes the transference of knowledge and the passing of the tradition from master to student.

Just as my master passed on his knowledge to me, it becomes the responsibility of my students to use what they have learned to enlighten their own lives. To this day, many of my students remain close to me. Some have even gone on to make martial arts their life by opening up schools of their own. Many eventually go their own way, of course, as they choose professions and settle down with their families. Somehow though, I always feel responsible for them all. I often wonder how many will continue with their training. I wonder how many will fulfill the true purpose of a martial artist by reaching that state of invincibility and humility in their lives. All I know is that I have given them the tools to do it.

The connection between master and student is an unbroken, undying one. I am reminded of an experience I had with my master some years ago. I was in Korea on a trip and decided to visit him. We hadn't seen each other for some time, but had always kept in touch. He was retired from teaching, but was still very active promoting Taekwondo and working with other masters. He was in his late seventies, but looked twenty years younger, full of health and vitality.

When we met, we bowed to each other, as is the custom in Korea. When I stood up again, I noticed that my master was still bowed and holding this position for some time. I thought to myself that I have been living in America so long, and that my bowing had become too quick. When he finally stood up, I saw in his eyes that his long bow had been out of deep respect for me.

He smiled and said, "Rhin Moon, you are fulfilling your destiny as a martial artist." I was speechless and could only smile back. His words meant the world to me, and the love I felt was deeper than the ocean.

By relaying my life story, I hope to show you the essence of what it means to become a martial artist.

It is my way of bowing to you.

(Rhin Moon) Richard Chun
New York City, 2002

Note to Readers:
Originally, Taekwondo was written as three words—Tae Kwon Do—to signify the meaning of each word, "Tae" meaning fist, "Kwon" meaning foot and "Do" meaning way. Many Korean Masters still write it this way. My previous books were written in this style. However, a present-day trend has been to write Tae Kwon Do as one word, particularly in references to organizations such as the Taekwondo Federation or Taekwondo Association. In this book, I have kept up with this trend of writing Taekwondo as one word.

Acknowledgements

In writing a book about your life, every experience and every person that you come into contact with truly plays a role in the formation of who you are and becomes part of the fabric of your life. Just as it was necessary to highlight certain experiences that related directly to my life as a martial artist, there are specific people that I must acknowledge. Without these people in my life this book would not have come into fruition.

Grandmaster Chong Soo Hong in Korea, Founder of Taekwondo Moo Duk Kwan, my first teacher, remains my inspiration and the ideal of a martial arts master.

Grandmaster Ki Whang Kim from Silver Spring, Maryland, one of my early teachers, for his endless encouragement and support.

Dr. Un Yong Kim, my sincere advisor and strong supporter, whose many achievements include President of World Taekwondo Federation, Executive Member of International Olympic Committee, and President of the Korean Olympic Committee, has inspired me throughout the years and encouraged me to open my first school.

I cannot fail to mention two of my earliest students whose honor was mine to teach. Frank Fuentes, my first student and black belt, who lost his life in Vietnam. He was like a friend and son to me. Joseph Hayes, another early student and one of the best martial artists I have ever trained, is now an assistant minister in Texas.

I also wish to thank all my present black belts and students whose desire to learn and pass on this tradition continues to inspire me.

To my loving wife, Kwang Hae Chun, and my children, Yong Taik and Kyung Mee, whose love and support has been the center of my life around which everything else revolves.

I would like to thank my co-author, Richard LaMarita, who worked closely with me in writing this book. His clear vision and his organizational, writing, and editing skills helped shape and direct this project.

Finally, I would like to thank all the members of the Taekwondo Association who have taken the tradition of this martial art into their hearts so that it lives forever.

THE WORLD TAEKWONDO FEDERATION (WTF)

5th Fl. Shinmunno Bldg., 238 Shinmunno 1st -ga, Jongro-gu, Seoul, Korea 110-061
Tel: +82 2 566 2505/557 5446   Fax: +82 2 553 4728
E-mail : wtf@unitel.co.kr   Website : www.wtf.org

Taekwondo originated in Korea over two thousand years ago and has developed into a traditional martial art with over 50 million practitioners in 161 nations worldwide. Additionally, while evolving into one of the most modern, popular sports in the international arena, it has demonstrated the ideals of the Olympic Movement, that of harmony and progress throughout the globe. This has become all the more evident since it inauguration as an official sport in the Sydney Olympic Games.

The fundamental motive of Taekwondo practice is to improve and maintain physical fitness and to nurture self-defense skills. However, the underlying philosophy of Taekwondo puts a great deal of emphasis on promoting mental qualities that cultivate concentration, self-control, bravery, and a deep appreciation for humanity.

Furthermore, by becoming familiar with the Oriental belief system from which Taekwondo stems, the practitioner will gain a better understanding of the moral foundation supporting the art.

It gives me great pleasure, therefore, to write this letter of recommendation for a book I am certain will act as a base for the development of Taekwondo as a world martial art as well as a sport. In his book *Taekwondo Spirit & Practice*, the author, Richard Chun, with outstanding humility and compassion, opens his past to all practitioners and demonstrates what is required to achieve not merely success but a high level of proficiency in the martial arts. Clearly, Dr. Chun's many accomplishments over the decades speak for themselves and it is obvious to me that by following his footsteps through the martial arts, Taekwondoists everywhere will be inspired by his life experiences.

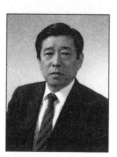

Dr. Un Yong Kim
Executive Board Member
International Olympic Committee
President
World Taekwondo Federation

CHAPTER 1

The Challenge

Class at the Moo Duk Kwan Institute always began with mopping the floor. This simple ritual served a dual purpose. The first was cleanliness. Soon, about 80 students—young twelve year old boys like myself to young men in their twenties—would be barefoot on that floor practicing the many hundred moves that comprised the art of Taekwondo. The second purpose was to instill in the novice a sense of pride and respect for our school and our art.

All of us at the school, excluding the black belts, were assigned to clean the floor in groups of five on a rotating basis. My turn came up about every ten days. When my time came around with four other students, I always arrived early. Grabbing a bucket and a mop, I quickly got out on the floor to clean off the sweat and marks from last night's matches and the dust that had settled during the night. When the others arrived, I usually had my section already done. I worked fast because I wanted to be first in the changing room and into my doboks.

Soon, all the students arrived and we were out on the floor warming up and practicing our forms. Our Master, Chong Soo Hong, emerged from his office about half an hour later to observe. He never said a word. He just stood off to the side in his crisp, white tobok with black trim, a black belt tied tightly around his waist and his face in deep concentration. He stood there with his arms crossed and expressionless for the longest time. Sometimes he clapped, indicating that he wanted our attention. We would immediately stop our practice, turn to face him, and bow. There was always a deafening silence.

Master Hong was a Grandmaster of the highest caliber. His teaching strictly followed traditional methods and his style was rigorous and disciplined. I was fortunate to be studying at his school as it was regarded as the best martial art school in Seoul in its day. I was fortunate in other ways though as well. I had the right start. It might not have been that way, however, if I had not learned the most fundamental lesson of the martial artist. That lesson took me six months to learn and went beyond mere mastery of technique. It is still deep within me like the memory of the sound of my master's voice. One afternoon, his voice broke the silence with words directed at me.

"Rhin Moon, please demonstrate for the class the turning hook kick." His voice echoed like a drum in the small gym.

"Yes, sir." I bowed respectfully.

Although many of these students had been studying Taekwondo much longer than I, our master had chosen me to demonstrate the kick. I stepped forward while the remaining students backed up towards the edges of the gym. I felt every eye upon me. My feet felt warm on the wood floor and my body felt strong and limber. All around me, the students in the class sat on the floor and watched in silence.

I had been studying for only two months at the institute. Our routine was the same and it was very demanding, precisely following the age-old tradition of the Taekwondo masters. Every few days, our master demonstrated a specific move to the students without taking any questions or giving any explanation. We simply observed. Our usual practice session, then, consisted of executing that move about two to three hundred times a day. Each move, according to tradition, must be drilled over and over again until it becomes second nature, like a part of your being. Only then would one gain the spontaneity, precision, and fluidity of form necessary to execute the move effectively and effortlessly in an actual combat situation. Our master would give the class an opportunity to ask questions only after he felt we had learned the basics of the move. Occasionally, however, he interrupted this routine to ask a student to demonstrate a specific punch or kick. It was an opportunity for him to informally test our progress. This was the first time I had been chosen.

I stood facing my master. My legs were spread apart, one foot in front of the other. I was slightly crouched to distribute my weight evenly and lower my center of gravity. My arms were raised in fighting position. Instinctively, I located a center of calm within as I prepared myself for the move. Like an arrow pulled back on the bow, I felt dynamic yet rested, still before the release. Then, with a burst of energy, I spun my upper body in the opposite direction of my imaginary opponent, my left leg following the motion. As I planted my left foot, my right leg sprung up and around for a hook kick to the head. In a fraction of a second, I resumed my original fighting stance.

I bowed again.

"Excellent demonstration," said Master Hong. He stood tall and upright with folded arms, his short hair oiled and parted on the side with not a single hair out of place. He rarely showed emotion. I admit that I was a bit afraid of him, yet that day, I thought I glimpsed a smile coming from his face. Not from his mouth, but in his eyes. Then, turning to address the class he added, "Rhin Moon is doing very well. Do as he does."

I returned to my position among the other students. Walking with my head down, I looked at my small feet and observed my own body—sinewy, muscular and agile. A few friends patted me on the back as I rejoined the group. I had performed well and I knew it. It was no surprise. I had been training hard and picking up new techniques quickly. Other students, who also noticed my progress, began to ask me for help during practice. I often demonstrated for a small group of two or three the finer points of maintaining a balanced stance during a kick, or how to twist the arm upward to deflect an incoming blow. Although I spent only three hours a day practicing at the institute, Taekwondo was quickly becoming my entire life. I thought of nothing else.

When practice was over that day, it was early evening and the streets of Seoul were teeming with people on trolleys and bicycles hurrying back to their homes. The walk from the Moo Duk Kwan Institute to my home in Bukahyun-Dong village was three miles, but the time passed quickly. I relived in my mind the demonstration I had performed in class that day, and the overcrowded streets soon faded from my view. It was clear to me that I was progressing quickly at the school and this was exactly what I wanted. I felt an intense purpose for being there, a purpose that only I had known. I had begun my practice of the martial arts solely to prepare myself to fight someone, and soon, I would be ready to do just that.

The incident had taken place in a playground after school one day. At that time, there were no organized sports in school for boys to compete in. Without such an outlet, we naturally created our own. Rivalries developed between boys from different schools and villages with competitions in running, soccer, and gymnastics held informally after school hours. Challenges were made on the sandlots, in the streets, at the marketplaces, at any time and to any group who would accept. I was proud to belong to the group from Bukahyun-Dong village. We were one of the best groups and often triumphed in our competitions.

Bukahyun-Dong was located in the northwest part of Seoul at the foot of the mountains. It was an upper class residential section with winding tree-lined streets and large homes. Doctors, lawyers, educators, and businessmen lived there. Numerous schools were located in Bukahyun-Dong and its neighboring village and there were several parks and recreational facilities. We were a group of a dozen headstrong boys who prided ourselves on our elite position.

I held the position of daejang in this group. Daejang is a term given to someone who is the leader, one who stands out. The literal meaning of daejang is major-general. To be daejang, you must show courage and strong will. Although I was not the smartest, biggest, or strongest among my friends, I exhibited this courage and was quite outspoken. One day our gang was gathered on the street and I challenged anyone to drop a match into a pothole where we placed some carbide which was used back then as a substitute for gasoline. Since no one accepted, I naturally did it, throwing a lit match into the hole. The carbide exploded, scorching my face and burning all my hair and eyebrows. It took me one month to heal and my parents were very upset with me, but I had become daejang. As daejang, I insisted on being in charge of all matters relating to our group. Since I thought that I was most often right in making decisions, I felt that anything I said should be immediately obeyed without question.

Not everyone agreed on this point, however, and for a while, a boy named Sang Keun Chung had been challenging me. He was a tall boy with long arms and legs. He was good at kicking a soccer ball, but he could not run very fast. At first, I ignored his challenges and forced my decision, but soon I started to become frustrated. One day we were gathered in a playground after school. A running competition was approaching and I began to inform everyone of the specific events they would be running. That's when Sang Chung jumped in.

"Why do I have to run that race? I don't want to. I want to run in the third race."

"You are not fast enough," I said. "And why are you always resisting me in decisions that I make. Why do you do this? I am the leader." We began to argue.

The other members of our group looked on as our words became more heated. We argued face to face, trying to break down each other's resistance, but we were getting nowhere. At that point, to bring this disagreement to a close, I shoved him, but even then, he did not give up. I approached again to intimidate him and to enforce my authority when, suddenly, he swung his fist and I was knocked down to the ground. He stood over me for a while and then walked away.

I picked myself up and looked to a friend. I was shaking like a leaf.

"Didn't you know," my friend said, "Sang Chung is studying boxing."

The rest of the group quickly dispersed and my position as daejang crushed. I had been disgraced, knocked over. I felt like a fallen king. What made matters worse was that I had not wanted to fight and I had not actually challenged Chung but suddenly, I was down and beaten. I felt deeply ashamed and lost face as the leader in my group.

Looking back at this incident, with a perspective from many years later, I see that an eleven-year-old boy with a bruised ego tends to make things bigger than they really are. But back then, for days afterward, I could not stop thinking about the fight. The incident plagued me, eating away at my peace of mind. I avoided seeing my friends, taking new routes home from school and riding my bicycle by myself. I had been the daejang, a position among my friends that I sought and valued, but I was reduced to just someone else, not strong enough to be a leader. I had never felt that way. My confidence was eroded, I began to lose concentration in my studies, and I felt uncomfortable even in my own home. Something had to be done; I had to regain my position as daejang. So, I decided to challenge Chung to fight.

I kept the plan to myself and thought it best to prepare for the challenge. I did not know how to fight and needed to learn. Since he was a boxer and knew how to punch, I did not want to fight him that way. So, I decided to study Tae Kwan Do (or Tang Soo Do as it was called then) because of its emphasis on kicking techniques. The Korean word "tae" means "to kick" or "squash with the foot," while "kwon" implies a "hand or fist to block and punch," and "do" means "the art" or "the way." Thus, literally translated, "Taekwondo" means "the art of kicking, blocking, and punching." This was the form of martial art in which I wanted to train in order to prepare myself for the challenge.

In finding a place to study Taekwondo, certain considerations were important. A school close to my home in Bukahyun-Dong village taught this form of martial art, but a few of my friends were studying there already and I wanted to train in secret. I had heard of another school, the headquarter school for this branch of martial art, three miles away in the downtown section of Seoul. I decided to visit it one day after school.

My first walk to the institute was long and lonely. The streets led through the business district of Seoul, past tall, unfriendly buildings with many people scurrying about, and downtown past the main railroad station. I walked through the open air market where vendors sold fruit and vegetables and other stands that sold lamps, pots and pans, vases, ink drawings, and sculptures. Down a long block a one-story square building sat on the corner. It was colorless with few windows. A wooden sign hung next to the door that read 'Moo Duk Kwan Institute.'

I walked in and stood inconspicuously along the wall. The building housed a small gym with a dull wooden floor. On a wall hung a large portrait of the master of the school, his face looked chiseled out of stone, strong and confident. It was flanked, on one side, with the Korean flag and, on the other side, a banner of a fist surrounded by branches with leaves. (I would soon learn that this banner was the Moo Duk Kwan emblem symbolizing the spreading of peace, justice, and human advancement throughout Korea and the world.) The students were dressed in doboks with different color belts. They were organized in distinct rows, executing the same move. There was a grace, power, and purity to their movements that felt like an ocean wave. It was silent except for the deep voice of the instructor, the squeak of their bare feet on the wooden floor, and an occasional yell by the students in unison that reverberated throughout the gym. I felt a stir of excitement well up inside my chest, and there and then, I decided to join. A little while later, I approached the master and signed up to start classes immediately.

Keeping my training a secret was a simpler matter than you might have expected. If my friends inquired, I simply told them that I had been working out with weights or riding my bicycle on my own. They seemed to accept this and pressed no further. Hiding it from my parents was a bit more complex. I could easily account for my time, but that time now cost money. I told them that our group was training for a track and field competition or soccer match and this seemed to satisfy them. However, I needed to raise money to cover the cost for my training. The weekly allowance that I received from my father was not quite enough. To supplement my allowance, I needed to take on a part-time job. I soon found one, believe it or not, right in my own home. My father actually became my new part-time employer.

Being a prominent doctor in Bukahyun-Dong village, my father would often come home after a full day's work with sore muscles, aches, and pains. I offered to massage him, knowing that he would increase my allowance. So, every evening on a small bed in the back room of our home, I massaged my father to pay for my expenses at the institute. There were times that I felt guilty for having this little secret, yet I never said anything and no questions were ever asked.

Everyday after school I would rush to the gym to learn new punches and kicks, drilling and executing these moves many times until they felt part of me. I was gaining strength, flexibility, and confidence day by day. I saw my progress only in terms of my fighting ability, and I saw myself using this art only to regain my position as daejang. I never lost sight of that purpose. The master and students at the institute, who noticed my progress and encouraged me to continue, had no inkling of my motive for learning with such fierce, single-minded determination.

During this time, there was little contact with my friends at school, except during class time. I did miss them, however, after classes during our playtime, and one day on my way home from the institute, I passed a park where I saw my old group playing soccer. In the distance, I watched them for a while and I felt sad. I noticed that Chung was the goalkeeper in the game and I saw him block a shot with his long arms and give instructions to his teammates where to run. I watched them until I thought I saw Sang Keun turn in my direction. I turned away and hurried home, hoping he didn't see me.

Time went by very quickly, and in six months, I had earned my green belt. I had also won some tournaments for my level and age group. These were fine achievements. But, more importantly to me, then, was that I felt ready to challenge Sang Keun. The day when I would regain my position as daejang was soon approaching. A few days later, I saw Sang Keun during school and asked him if he would meet me afterwards. I said that I wanted to speak to him about something. He was not aware of my intentions and agreed. I felt sure of myself and ready for the challenge. I wanted to seek revenge on him and show the group that if it was necessary to fight to be daejang, I would do it.

After school, that day, he was waiting for me with the other members of our group just off the school grounds.

"Hello, Sang Keun," I said.

"Hello, Rhin Moon. I have been waiting for you."

"Yes, let's walk and I will tell you."

Sang Keun and I began walking down the road that led to our village. I enjoyed seeing my friends; some crowded around me asking what I had been doing. Others walked beside Sang Keun. No one knew I had been training in the martial arts. They were unsure why I had wanted to meet with them. When we were far enough from the school grounds, I turned and faced Sang Keun with a very angry expression on my face. I was trembling and my fists were clenched.

"You knocked me down before," I said with a husky, angry voice, "and now I am ready to fight you. I want to challenge you." With these words I prepared myself for his attack.

Out of the group, one of the boys yelled, "Rhin Moon, what are you doing? Are you crazy? Sang Keun is now the leader." The others backed away to see what would happen.

At first, Sang Keun looked angry and curled his hands into fists. But what he did next astounded me.

He dropped his fists and said, "I cannot accept your challenge. I hit you before because you were pushing me. It was sudden. I didn't even mean it. I am sorry for what happened at that time."

"You give up?" I responded.

"No. You are a good leader. If you want to be daejang, you can be daejang. Only, sometimes, I don't want to do everything you say. I want to do other things. If you want, you can hit me now" he said, and then he closed his eyes.

I couldn't believe what I heard. In the presence of my friends, again, I felt shame wash over me, but this time—six months later and with a green belt in Taekwondo—it stung even more deeply. Yet, along with the shame, I felt humbled.

"You have knocked me down again," I said. "Let's be friends." I extended my hand in friendship. He took it. Then, I turned to the group.

"I have been studying Taekwondo at another school, hiding it from you. I am sorry. You are my friends."

Then, I had a thought and looked towards downtown. "I must see my master." I turned and ran as fast as I could all the way to the institute, feeling the fear that I had for Master Hong increase as I drew nearer, feeling the fear I had for him dissipate for what I must do. I entered the school well before the practice session. No one was there except for Master Hong, sitting in his office, reading and drinking tea.

"Master Hong, I must talk to you, please."

I bowed, sweat running off my forehead. My feet were hot and dusty. His face looked gentle like a father.

"Master Hong, I did something wrong. I challenged my friend to fight. I wanted to beat him. He punched me and I've been angry, all this time. I've been training here just to fight him. Now, I don't know if I can train anymore. I don't feel worthy."

My mind was in a whirl.

"Rhin Moon, Rhin Moon, calm down," said Master Hong. "You are one of my best students." His gaze was penetrating, yet warm and friendly. I did not feel scared of him anymore.

"But you should never enter the study of the martial arts to seek revenge," he said. "It is an honor and responsibility to train in this tradition. We are not here solely to become fighters. Our purpose is not to be an instrument of violence, but rather an instrument of peace."

I didn't understand his words and said, "I don't know if I can continue my studies. I have been angry and. . . ."

Master Hong would not even let me finish the sentence. He leaned over and placed his cup of tea on the table. It smelled of jasmine.

"You must learn to think before you act, and not be impulsive," he said. "The action of a martial artist is like flowing water, Rhin Moon."

I held my head down in shame, but when he called my name, I looked up at him and listened to his words.

"Water is destructive if it flows with unleashed power and fury. It can uproot trees and carry away rocks like corks. Or water can be constructive if it flows with grace and ease. It bends and courses in the simplest way through a field or forest. In both cases, the goal is met; the water flows to the sea. You can be fierce and furious, or graceful and easy in your actions. To act with grace and dignity is simpler, Rhin Moon, and even more powerful. Now, get changed, you are late for practice."

"Yes, sir," I said, and bowed many times, almost unconsciously and awkwardly, before him.

A few days later, it was my turn to mop the floor. I arrived early, as usual, but that time even much earlier than the other students who were also expected to help. I pulled out the mop and bucket, and by myself, I cleaned the entire floor. When the other students arrived, they saw the job was completely done.

"Look, Rhin Moon has mopped the floor for us," one boy said.

"He is becoming a martial artist," I heard another say.

Thinking back upon this experience, I realize how lucky I was. If my challenge to fight had been met, I probably would have won very easily. In the gloating of that victory, my desire for revenge would have been fulfilled, yet in reality, I would have been the loser. Using martial arts solely as a means for self-defense would have served its purpose and I probably would have felt satisfied enough to end my training. Instead, from this experience, I saw that I had much to learn. I realized, then, that the martial arts are a way of life and not a way of fighting. Even at my young age, I saw the enormous depth and philosophy in it that I did not know existed before, and I realized that within the practice and training of the forms was a life work and an understanding of which to aspire and attain.

Yes, I was lucky because an experience that could have easily ended my life as a martial artist fatefully began it. The challenge that I offered to my friend ironically turned itself upon me, challenging me with the words that I would say to myself over and over: "Don't be satisfied with being merely a fighter. Become a martial artist."

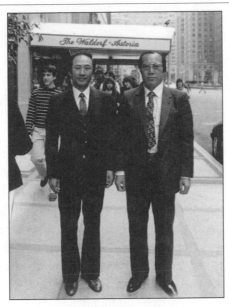

With Grandmaster and Vice President of Kukkiwon, Chong Soo Hong, New York, 1970's.

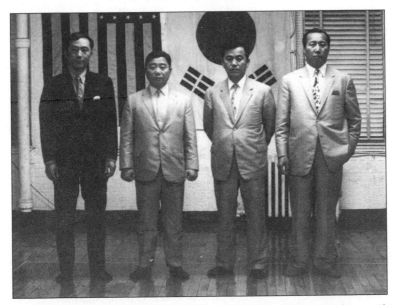

With the past presidents of Moo Duk Kwan. Left to right; Richard Chun, Grandmaster Chang Yong Chung, Grandmaster Kang Ik Lee, Grandmaster Ching Soo Hong 1970's.

CHAPTER 2
The Peak of Hallasan

They were three days of eternity. Three never-ending days of waiting. The test for black belt was over and I could do nothing now except wait. Years of hard work lay behind me. My life as a martial artist lay before me, and yet it all seemed to come down to a sheet of paper posted on the small corkboard that hung on a wall at the Institute. I had seen it all before during the previous black belt tests—the nervousness and anxiety in my fellow student's faces, the single sheet that announced if your years of training had come to fruition, the jostling before the posted results searching to find your name, the explosion of relief and happiness when you found it, the turning away in dejection and disappointment if you did not. Those three days of waiting to see if I had passed the test to earn my black belt seemed to pass even more slowly than the three years of training it took to get to that point.

I felt confident during the test, performing all the forms and breaks in a smooth, accomplished manner. No obvious mistakes were made. Still, there were three judges to convince. They sat silently, expressionless, behind a long table at the end of the gym and observed the forty candidates for black belt. In two groups of twenty, our instructor led us through a demonstration of advanced forms. My execution of the forms was impeccable, I thought. I had trained hard and often taught these same moves to students who progressed slower than I. Then, we moved on to breaking techniques. With classmates holding the boards, two students at a time performed before the judges. I executed a hop sidekick, flying sidekick, and double punch, breaking 3 boards with each move. The test concluded with a minute of non-contact free fighting.

I tried to ease my worry during those three days by telling myself that everything would turn out as it should. It was out of my hands at this point, yet I was so preoccupied with the anticipation of knowing the results that a constant nervousness churned in my stomach during the waiting period. I was edgy and did not sleep well. When I entered the Institute on the third day and saw a group of boys crowded before a notice on the corkboard, immediately I felt some sense of relief. The time had come. The results had been posted. I made my way through the crowd, straining my neck to catch a glimpse of the names. They were listed in alphabetical order. I scanned the names, my heart racing like a tightly wound clock. Kim, Dock Man—Kim, Keum Soo—Chun, Rhin Moon. (In the Korean alphabet, the letter 'K' comes before the letter 'C'). There it was. Halfway down the column. I saw my name written in clear, block letters. I had made it. I had earned my black belt. I walked away feeling fulfilled, giving congratulations to other friends who had also passed, receiving pats on my back. It was surely one of the happiest days in my life and a feeling of great accomplishment swelled within me, culminating the next day in a beautiful ceremony that was given in honor of the new black belts.

I had never seen the Institute look so beautiful before. Banners with inspiring messages in elegant calligraphy draped the walls of the gym. A small platform with sprays of flowers and a podium was set up. Many dignitaries and special guests including town politicians, community leaders, and families of the black belt recipients, were present. My family had come to share in my accomplishment. Seats in the front two rows were reserved for the new black belts. As we entered in single file dressed in our doboks with the emblem of our Institute on our chest everyone stood and applauded. The sound echoed and reverberated throughout the gym. I felt so proud. The Grand Master and Head of the Institute, Master Chong Hong, began the ceremonies with an inspiring speech. I remember his words even to this day.

"The black belt is an honor that you will carry with you the rest of your lives," he said. "To attain this honor required skill and expertise in numerous fighting techniques. It is a physical achievement of strength, stamina, conditioning, and coordination of the highest degree. Yet, a black belt represents much more than just a physical achievement."

He paused as if he were contemplating revealing an intimate secret. Then, he continued.

"A black belt means that you have completed the first step to becoming a master of the martial arts," he said directing his gaze at us, "and a master of the martial arts is nothing less than a master of the self."

Master Hong continued talking about this deeper and more profound meaning of the black belt, explaining that the inner strength and self-confidence that comes to us from this art applies not only to the field of the martial arts, but wherever our future life takes us. I remember listening intently to his words, understanding them as words, understanding their concept, but at the age of fourteen, not really grasping the full impact of their meaning. That would take me a lifetime. He went on to praise the determination that we exhibited in our endeavor to achieve the black belt and, then, proudly announced our names and tied our new black belt individually around our waists.

In the tradition of Taekwondo, it is a custom when a student receives his or her black belt that a master ties the belt around your waist for the first time to symbolize the passing of the tradition from master to student. When Master Hong tied the crisp, new belt around my waist I felt as if an electric current passed between us. Wearing the black belt around my waist for the first time made me feel like part of an elite club. I kept on tightening it, and wore it for the longest time even when the day's celebration was over. I didn't want to take it off.

At the end of the ceremony, Master Hong again spoke, looking directly at each one of us seated before him.

"Now, as new black belts, it is your responsibility to be pure representatives of this art and, through your leadership, to pass this knowledge to the next generation."

Even at the age of fifteen, that thought thrilled me and brought a sense of peace and order into my life. I wanted to live that ideal. My sense of self, my admiration of my family, my behavior with my friends, at that time, all pointed to a boy enticed with the idea of leadership, of bringing positive values into people's lives, and striving for the highest that human nature can achieve. I knew that I had the makings of an enlightened leader inside of me and I yearned to become a great martial artist. Our Grand Master's speech that afternoon crystallized these feelings for me and brought my development as a martial artist, that day, to a higher level.

There are universal values in human nature—inner strength, a positive self-image, a strong moral character—that when sufficiently developed in an individual keep one's life always in an evolutionary direction. The study of Taekwondo, although a highly focused discipline of physical excellence, transcends itself to develop these universal values in life. These values develop side by side with the mastery of specific forms and fighting techniques through hard work, patience, experience, and study. To become a true martial artist, you must be aware of the completeness of the tradition and philosophy and develop both these inner and outer aspects. I was very fortunate because that seed was planted inside of me during my early years of training. Throughout my life, it has grown into a tree that bears a beautiful fruit, but like any plant or tree, it requires proper care and nourishment. The work is never done.

The next couple of years of my life after earning my black belt were highly productive. With this heightened understanding of the role of the martial artist, I expanded my activities with the institute. I continued training, refining my skills as a black belt, attending local tournaments sponsored by branches of the Institute that were established in towns outside of Seoul. However, most importantly, I became involved in the training of new and intermediate students at these branch institutes. Through my contacts and teaching, I made many friends and felt as if I were putting into action what our Grand Master spoke about at the ceremony. I gained the respect and admiration of many people through my activities during this time, and I felt that I was truly becoming a true martial artist and leader.

In the midst of these happy years, the Korean War suddenly broke out and put an end to it all.

It happened like the sudden shot of a gun. Government officials assured the citizens of Seoul that relations between the South and North were cordial. In reality however, the North Koreans had long been threatening the South. On June 25, 1950, North Korea invaded and war broke out. Within three days, the invading North Korean forces had almost reached Seoul. Government spokesmen told its people not to worry, that it could defend itself against the North. But the next day, North Korean soldiers captured Seoul and the South Korean government quickly fled south. The retreating South Korean forces destroyed the Han River Bridge to prevent the Northern military army from following. In doing so however, they also made it impossible for the citizens of Seoul to escape. Overnight, Seoul turned from a peaceful, bustling city into a chaotic battleground. Fighting broke out in the streets with guns, tanks, and smoke bombs. Buildings were burned and destroyed and many people were killed.

Our family was suddenly thrust into danger. We were warned that upper class families should be particularly careful. My father, a prominent citizen of Seoul and the President of the Doctor's Association, would be killed if the communists caught him. Without any warning, our lives were being swept out from under us. I feared for my father, my family, and for myself. Friends I knew had been drafted and, years later, I learned many had been killed. I did not want to fight, and luckily, I could not since I was just one year under the cut-off age. I simply wanted to get away from the war as our family had done before during World War II. Soon, as fate would have it, my wish would be fulfilled.

To protect us, my father closed his medical practice and decided to take our family, temporarily, to the port city of Inchun. We would stay there for a while to see if the fighting subsided. As a precaution, however, my father bought a junk boat in Inchun with two other families in the event that we needed to flee even farther from the war. If necessary, we would sail to Cheju Island off the southern tip of Korea. A few weeks later General MacArthur landed at Inchun with the United States troops. The momentum seemed to be turning in our direction. We hurried back to Seoul in the hopes that the American presence would quickly resolve the conflict. It did, but unfortunately, for only a short period of time. In the winter of 1951, the North Koreans again drove south, and the war escalated. My father knew what had to be done.

One evening, he announced, "This war is not letting up. There is nothing left to do. Tomorrow night, we are sailing to Cheju Island. I have made all the arrangements." I knew the decision that my father made was the right one, but still my first thought was if I would ever see Seoul again. I didn't know and, with the upheaval and uncertainty of the time and my life all seeming to come crashing down, I cried.

The following evening we sailed out of Inchun harbor. We made our escape as a cold, winter wind whipped through the bay muffling the deep sounds of the boat's engines. Below deck, I huddled with my brothers and sisters in a musty room lit only with a single light bulb. Wearing an oversized sweater and coat, I was cold and scared. The boat creaked and rocked as it made its way out to the open sea. Two other families were on the boat with us. No one spoke. We just all stared at each other, wondering what would become of us. Questions flooded my mind. Would I ever see my home and friends again? What was going to happen to my life? Could I continue my martial arts training without a master? Was I ready to be a martial artist on my own? Fear swirled with confusion and anger deep inside of me until I drifted off to sleep, gently rocked by the boat.

Today, a vacation to Cheju Island by boat takes half a day. In 1951, it took three families three weeks in a battered, small boat to reach the island. About halfway through our voyage, the boat's engine sputtered and died out, leaving us free-floating on a windless sea for a couple of days. When the wind finally picked up, the navigator set a course again, steering the ship to a nearby island. For a few days, my father exchanged medical services for repairs on the ship and enough provisions to reach Cheju. We left the island as soon as repairs were completed and resumed our voyage. About a week later on a sunny day, we sailed into the small harbor of Cheju City.

Cheju is a large volcanic island that lies 50 miles off the southern tip of the mainland. The island is rimmed by a serene coastline of rock and beaches. Plains and valleys of lush subtropical vegetation stretch inland where wild horses graze and farmers grow wheat and beans. At the geographical center, like a mighty god overlooking the entire island, Mt. Hallasan rises up over 6,000 feet. A magnificent mountain, with its peak often hidden in mist and cloud cover, Mt. Hallasan is always in the islander's awareness and imagination.

In the early 1950's, over 50,000 natives populated the island. They were concentrated mainly in and around its main city on the north shore, Cheju City. During the war however, thousands of families made their way to Cheju Island, inundating the simple, peasant way of life with mainland sophistication and problems. These families lived an upper class life on the mainland since only the wealthiest could afford to get to Cheju at that time. They considered themselves elite and were accustomed to a high standard of living. The transition to life as a refugee was difficult for them to say the least. Jobs were scarce, food was scarce, and living conditions were far below what they were accustomed to. Most of the refugees lived in tents on a mountainside outside of Cheju City where housing was crude and cramped. Many refugee families supported themselves at the open-air market, selling commodities imported from the mainland, particularly foods and clothing. My father, however, set up a small medical practice for the refugees and native population. That allowed us to rent a small cottage on a hillside outside the city.

Our house was simple and rustic. There were four small rooms made of rock and earthen walls. There was no plumbing, sparse lighting, and it was covered with a thatched roof. Due to the strong winds that often hit the island, the roof had to be tied down with straw ropes and logs piled on top for added security. The house, however, was one of the nicer ones on the island for a refugee family. It also afforded a view of Cheju City to the front. In the back Mt. Hallasan loomed in the distance.

Cheju Island is very beautiful. The weather is tropical and breezy in the warmer months, and lush and sunny all year round. Often, I would walk alone into the hills surrounding the city. In the quiet fields of grass with Mt. Hallasan in view, I began to practice my martial art forms by myself. It was all that I brought with me to Cheju Island. In Seoul, I left behind my friends and my master. I did not know if I would ever see them or train officially in the martial arts again. Yet, I found that the knowledge of the forms lived on within me. However, without a master to watch over me and correct my mistakes, training on my own demanded even more discipline and concentration than ever before because I didn't want to create bad habits or learn incorrect techniques. As a result, I was forced to keep my mind and body completely focused and coordinated when I trained.

I learned very clearly during this time that Taekwondo is truly an art and not just a sport. In the martial arts, unlike other sports, you do not need fancy equipment or a pair of the latest sneakers to train properly. You simply need the desire to work hard and keep your mind and body integrated as one and focused on your goal. It took every ounce of energy and concentration for me during this time to train all by myself. I still felt the knowledge was silent and hidden deep inside of me like the peak of Mt. Hallasan—always hidden in mist and clouds.

I trained as often as I could whenever I was not in school. I attended a high school specifically designed for the refugees, which was located in a playground in Cheju City. More than 500 students were cramped under a large open-air tent, without enough desks and exposed to the wind and cold. Most of our life revolved in and around the school and the playground. Interaction between the natives of the island and the refugees was kept to a minimum, yet it was inevitable. We were looked down upon by the islanders who attended a larger school nearby. Although their school, a simple two-story structure, would have been considered a small one in Seoul, it seemed like a palace in comparison to our tent. We were envious of them. But, that was the least of our problems. The islanders hardly accepted or welcomed us on the island. They felt as if we were invading their island and not the ones who had fled from being invaded. There was a cultural distance between us that seemed impossible to cross.

The islanders were a simple people and proud of their heritage. They did not open their hearts easily to outsiders. Their main occupations were farming, fishing, and diving for shellfish and seafood. They wore colorful clothing of blues, reds, and yellows. Our presence on Cheju Island meant an inevitable change in their way of life. Our tastes and style of dress were different and we brought an influx of new foods, products, and ideas. They were either unwilling or unable to make the change and, as a result, tension between them and us grew, and incidents of verbal harassment began to occur frequently. I had managed to steer clear of any problems, spending my time either at school or in the mountains practicing my forms.

Soon, however, the refugees discovered that I had trained in the martial arts. Since I happened to be the only one, they asked me to defend them from the islanders. Of course, I flatly refused. I told them it was a ridiculous request. Like the war on the mainland, I did not want to get involved. My life had been interrupted already. Now, I simply wanted to live here without any problems and train on my own. Besides, what could I do to bridge such a large gap between two different peoples? These were my feelings. I was adamant about them. However, I had to admit to myself that I also heard a voice within me that said I should defend the refugees against what is wrong. If a martial artist is supposed to be a defender of justice and leader of people, according to tradition, then I must follow that principle. It is my responsibility, as Master Hong had instructed. However, for the moment, I did nothing.

One day, when my sister and some of her friends had been threatened on a walk through the city, that voice within me had to speak out. My training in the martial arts had instilled within me too deep a sense of responsibility and loyalty to turn away from a situation that was not right. I could not turn away any longer. I would not be confrontational and I would avoid fighting at all cost. I had been taught that as a martial artist resorting to physical force is the last option. I am an instrument of peace and order Master Hong taught me, I reminded myself. I decided to simply have a talk with the islanders.

A few days later I walked to the high school that the islanders attended. Classes would be let out soon, so I waited near a gate where the students would exit. They soon approached. I noticed that many of them were carrying small hand tools, such as shovels, rakes, hoes, and clippers, since the school specialized in agricultural classes. Seeing so many students with potential weapons put me on my guard, and I wondered if coming here to defend the refugees on my own was a wise move. The students saw me and stopped. Then, one boy stepped out from the crowd and asked what I wanted from them.

"There has been too much harassment between the people on this island

and the refugees," I said. "I just want to ask you to stop."

"Then, why don't you leave," someone yelled out from the crowd. "Why are you here? We didn't ask you to come."

"You don't understand. We have been forced to leave the mainland. We have been forced to give up our homes and way of life due to the war. We did not want to leave, but we were forced to. We don't want to give you problems. We don't want any problems. But, if you continue to threaten us, we must defend ourselves."

Then, to my surprise, I added, "If you must challenge us, then challenge me. Do it now if you want."

I don't know exactly why I said this, maybe to show off, maybe I thought I could end this problem right then and there with one simple action. I almost regretted saying it, knowing that I shouldn't have acted impulsively, yet I did say it. So, I waited for a response.

There was silence and no one approached or made a move. My words surprised and shocked them. This was something new to the islanders. No one had come up to them and stood up for their rights. I realized, then, that they were an untouched and pure people. I was actually moved by their response and, in fact, felt an immediate liking to them. Without another word, I parted and the peace had been maintained. The story of my challenge soon spread to all the children of the refugees, and I immediately became a hero and leader. I became a kind of defender of the refugees—a title that I didn't really want.

The harassments died down for a while. Then, about two weeks later, I received word through a friend that I should meet some islanders in their schoolyard at a certain time and day. I debated with myself for a few days whether I should tell anyone or ask for help, but I decided I would go alone. A few days later, I went to the schoolyard. Six boys were waiting for me.

As I approached they asked, "Why are you causing trouble?"

"I am not causing trouble," I responded. "I'm only defending our rights."

These six boys were older than I, and I felt they were not here to talk. We stood facing each other for a while, one looking at six. I began to sense danger and immediately became very alert, knowing that I had to make the first move.

"If someone wants to challenge me, you can do it one at a time or all together," I said.

There was no response. Knowing that if six boys attacked at the same time it would be a dangerous situation, I made some simple motions in the direction of one boy, and everyone dispersed, running away in different directions. The confrontation ended and again the story spread. This time though, I knew it was not over.

I waited to see what would come without asking for any assistance. Then, one day while walking home from school soon after the incident, two Cheju Island government officials approached me. They wanted to ask me a few questions and escorted me to a small building in the city. As we entered the door, another man was waiting, seated behind a desk.

"Please sit down," he instructed. I hesitated, but seeing that two men were standing behind me and he in front of me, I really didn't have any choice.

He began to talk explaining about life on the island. Then, he said something about me "causing problems and dissension between the refugees and the islanders." I began to answer strongly, and without warning, was suddenly struck in the head by one of the men behind me and also hit in the face by the man in front of me. I became scared. These men were much older and stronger than I. I realized that I had gotten myself too deeply into this without any help. I wondered why I thought that I could solve such a large problem on my own, but now it was too late to back down. I had to remain calm, without getting defensive or showing my fright.

"This is untrue. I am trying to resolve the conflict between us, not cause it," I said.

"Then, why do you challenge our people," they said.

"I am only standing up for our rights ... "

"What rights?" interrupted one of the men behind me.

"To live here," I said. "We cannot leave. Our lives have been changed because of this war and so must yours. We must find a way to live peacefully together."

They were listening. I knew that I could not defend myself in this situation through any show of force whatsoever. If these were government officials, they had abused their power by striking me. My only hope was to be balanced in my inner being, strong in my convictions, and truthful in my words.

In ancient history, Korea was a divided territory of three ruling kingdoms each often fighting independently the attack of foreign aggressors. Taekwondo emerged from centuries of bitter struggles and wars as a means to maintain our cultural integrity through its philosophical roots and as a means of national defense to fight off foreign domination through its use of fierce fighting techniques. The basic principles of Taekwondo were the pillars upon which it stood and which are still being taught in the best martial art schools today. These principles are responsibility, sincerity, and justice. One must develop these attitudes in their life to go hand in hand with the mastery of physical forms and techniques. While on Cheju Island, I realized how deeply I had imbibed these principles in myself. While working on my fighting forms far away from home, far away from my master, I saw that I already possessed within me the essence of this great tradition. I realized also the power of this silent, inner aspect of Taekwondo. It was, in fact, the strongest weapon that I used in my dealing with the problem between the islanders and refugees, and I had used it intuitively and spontaneously.

The men let me go. I went home and immediately told my father what had happened. He reported the incident to other government officials and discovered that what had happened to me had not been authorized. The three men were reprimanded and penalized for their actions. The government of Cheju City apologized to my father. However, the most important outcome was that all harassment stopped after this, and a real understanding seemed to take hold within the minds of the people of Cheju Island and the refugees. A bridge, albeit a simple one, had been built between us.

My reputation as a leader spread. I was known as the young one on the island who helped to defend the refugees and bring peace between the islanders and the refugees. For me, I knew that my show of strength and integrity came from inside me in the most natural and spontaneous manner. I didn't plan it in any way. In my training, a sense of fearlessness, defending right from wrong, and a love of truth had quietly developed and remained alive, even if I were far away from my homeland and master. Like a deep spark that had been hidden, it was ignited only by the circumstances of my life there. I remembered the words of my master who said that becoming a master of the martial arts would benefit us outside the realm of martial arts. Martial artists become leaders by mastering themselves. This is what had taken place for me on Cheju Island.

I continued my training in the hillsides near Cheju City. One day was particularly sunny with a gentle breeze in the air, and at one point while working on my forms, I happen to glance up and notice that the clouds on Mt. Hallasan, for that instant, had cleared and the snow-covered peak was visible.

CHAPTER 3
Tactics and Techniques

Seoul, Korea, 1954. I was 19 years old. Along with many thousands of refugees, I had returned to Seoul after the war to rebuild my life. During the final year of the war, I had enrolled at Yonsei University, a Christian college in Seoul that had relocated to Pusan, the second largest city in the south of Korea. When the war finally ended, the university moved back to its campus in Seoul and I followed, planning to major in economics and history so I could enter the business field upon graduation. It was a creative time for myself and for all Koreans. Everyone worked hard to re-establish themselves. The city itself was rebuilding: new office buildings, hotels, and residences were under construction, roadways were repaved, businesses and schools reopened. A sense of freedom and happiness—a natural feeling after an experiencing war—permeated life in Seoul.

I returned to the home in Bukahyun-Dong village that our family had left before the war. I lived with two of my brothers and one sister, who also returned to Seoul to resume their studies. The remainder of my siblings had stayed on Cheju Island to finish their schooling and live with my parents, who had also decided to remain. During the war, my father had established his medical practice and had become a prominent doctor and citizen of Cheju City much as he was in Seoul before the war. Their eldest children, however, were eager to get back to Seoul to fulfill their dreams. As always, my parents were supportive of our desires, and gave us the freedom to make our own decisions. They encouraged us to succeed and generously provided the means for our comfort. While in Seoul my father sent us a check every month to cover expenses, and if there was any remainder we divided between ourselves for entertainment.

I was particularly excited to be in Seoul again to resume martial arts training with established masters and black belts. However, I quickly discovered that the Moo Duk Kwan Institutes were not yet opened since the old masters needed time to re-establish their schools as they trickled back to Seoul. Old friends I trained with were now either gone or dispersed, some killed during the war, others residing elsewhere. The only contacts I had were a few known black belts currently attending Yonsei University. So I gathered them together and we began to train informally in the university cafeteria during off hours. It was the only space available to us.

Early morning or late afternoon, we would push the tables and chairs against the walls and practice forms, techniques, and sparring on the hard cafeteria floor. Often, a student would come into the cafeteria in anticipation of having a quiet, peaceful meal with some study time only to discover the space completely unusable. Needless to say, we didn't last long there! We were soon asked to discontinue our training due to the disturbance and inconvenience we were causing. The university could not supply us with an adequate space. They were sorry, and suggested that we look at the open-air theater on campus. It was unused, needed some repair, and might serve our purpose until they were more organized to allocate space for "official university clubs." That next day, we ventured out to explore the theater.

The open-air theater stood amid a grove of fir trees about 10 minutes walking distance from the main campus. It was built of stone and earth and resembled a Greek amphitheater, but with an Asian feel. Before the war, it was used to assemble the entire student body of Yonsei University for guest speakers, lecturers, and entertainment. At one end of the theater, a wood and earth stage had been set up, which would provide a place where we could train. It was in disrepair so we spent a day fixing some boards and leveling the earth, creating an outdoor gymnasium. It was not perfect, however. Although the space was private and cooled by the surrounding trees, rainy weather resulted in mud and slipperiness, making it impossible for us to practice. Nevertheless, the theater became our training center for the next six months.

We were a group of twenty at the start. After school hours, we met at the theater to review techniques and refine each other's moves. It was exhilarating to be working with others again. Our desire to develop as martial artists was reignited as we had missed the benefit of working together during the war. We had also missed the thrill of competition. Thus, the majority of our time during training was spent sparring. Out of this constant sparring, challenges arose and we came up with the idea to hold tournaments within our group. These tournaments became our incentive to progress. We learned to spar with martial artists of different styles and to work within a healthy atmosphere of competition.

We also became good friends very quickly, exchanging stories of our days during the war, discussing plans for the future, and socializing in the evenings. During this time, western ballroom dancing was very popular among the Korean people. It is an activity that I enjoy even to this day! Young people would meet in friend's homes or school gymnasiums in the evenings to dance the tango, waltz, or jitterbug. Often, after an evening out at the concert hall or a restaurant, we met at my house to dance because there was a large room on the first floor perfectly suited for dancing. My brothers and sister with their circle of friends would often join us.

Life was good. The war was over and I was very happy. Yet, during these times, I was keenly aware of an inner voice that told me that I was at a major turning point in my life. I felt a separation between old and new with respect to the times, my family, and my life. I thought a lot about it. Often as I walked down the streets of Bukahyun-Dong, I felt and saw the change. Children played soccer in the playgrounds and people shopped at the food markets. It was the same life I remember having nine years ago when I was a child. However, now I recognized no one and every face was new.

Even the house that I grew up in as a child, two buildings away from the one we lived in now, was always reminding me of coming change. Three buildings stood on the street, each a beautiful three-story structure. Before the war, our family lived in one and my father's offices and medical practices were in another. The third was a building solely for hospital beds. After the war, no one lived there. Seeing these buildings brought back many memories. I saw myself and my brothers and sisters playing as children. I heard our laughter and our crying. Our life had certainly been a privileged one. We were members of a prominent and wealthy family of Seoul. These streets that I once played in were my world. From these buildings my life had flowed from simple, innocent child-like desires. Now, it seemed everything was different and much more complicated.

My father and mother raised us as Christians with much kindness and love. We were a close-knit family with strong family values. My father worked long, hard hours and my mother ran a household and cared for a family of six boys and two girls. We were given the freedom to express ourselves and to be who we wanted. Discipline was enforced only when necessary. The only family rule that carried throughout the years was being home by ten o'clock. Although we were a close family, each of us had our own interests and circle of friends. I was always absorbed in athletics and physical activities, growing up a strong boy in body and mind. Whatever I decided to accomplish, I succeeded at it. We supported each other as we were doing again after the war, living together, linked together, yet keeping our own individuality. This was the atmosphere—one of love, comfort, freedom, and support—that I grew up in. This was my world. Then, larger forces—political and social ones—beyond our control changed everything. The first was in 1944 during World War II.

We had weathered the war untouched for four years until the spring of '44. We were alerted that the United States Air Force might bomb Seoul to rid the city of the Japanese. Fear gripped the city. We had heard of the death and destruction in the cities in Europe caused by air raids. My father wanted no part of this and wasted no time. He sold the three buildings that comprised our home and the hospital and we fled up north to my mother's hometown of Annack in the Hwang Hae Do province. We lived there in a small cottage near my mother's sister. My father used the money he made from selling our home and the hospital to buy some nearby land on a beautiful hillside. We would build our new home there if necessary, he said. About nine months later, we moved north to the capital city Pyung Yang and my father's hometown. We would wait there to see the outcome of the war. My father began to see patients, but only family and friends of family—nothing official.

Then, on August 15, 1945 the war suddenly ended. The U.S. had liberated Korea from Japanese rule. Japan had surrendered due to the total devastation of two cities caused by a new bomb. We were headed back to Seoul where my father bought our present house only two doors away from our original home in Bukahyun-Dong. His idea was to keep the land up north for vacation and maybe to move someday.

That idea quickly proved fruitless when the 38th parallel was drawn, dividing Korea into two distinct countries. Most of my father's and mother's families fled south and we lost everything that was left up north, including that beautiful patch of land on the hillside.

Being with my brothers and sister in Seoul after the Korean War was comforting, and I felt much gratitude towards my parents for bringing us up with such strong family values and ties, despite the major upheavals we faced. Our lives certainly had been strong and happy together. Now the war was over and we were beginning to branch out as all families must do. My parents moved to Cheju Island where they would remain for the rest of their lives. My brothers and sister would soon graduate college and begin their separate lives. What would life bring me? Where would it take me? These were only some of the many questions I asked myself at that time. I had no answers. Only time would tell.

I spent many of my hours studying the history of the Taekwondo tradition. This was a time of great inner development, a strengthening and rebuilding of myself, much like the city of Seoul. I drew upon my studies and experiences as a student of the Taekwondo tradition. It was important for me to develop a strong philosophical base because for the first time in my life, I realized that I would soon be out on my own. I wanted to be strong inside as well as outside for whatever the future would bring. The ten creeds of Taekwondo helped me fulfill this need. They were a source of great meaning and strength.

The ten creeds date back to the sixth century in Korean history, the Silla Dynasty, when a Buddhist monk named Won-Kwang formulated the creeds in his "Five Commandments." Won-Kwang was a man of great wisdom who dedicated his life to study and service. He became the personal advisor to the king in all spiritual matters. Young warriors also sought him out for instruction in behavioral codes thus creating a philosophical link to Taekwondo. His five commandments became the code of conduct for a group of warriors very much like the Knights of the Round Table in England, called the Hwarang-Do.

The history of the Hwarang-Do actually begins in the middle of the sixth century when King Chinhung created an order of young noblemen who would be potential leaders of the country. Scholars of Korean history have sought connections between Korea and China during this time. They believe that the Hwarang-Do actually has its origins in the code of Confucian ethics and the principles of Chinese military strategy of Sun Tzu, author of the now-famous treatise, *The Art of War.*

The Hwarang-Do emphasized the complete development of the person. This meant strong moral conduct, an appreciation of the arts, a love of learning, closeness to nature, and skill in the art of fighting. The actual word "Hwarang" is composed of the two words "Hwa" meaning flower and "Rang" meaning young master. In this time of Korean history, the flower symbolized glory, beauty, and integrity. So, "Hwarang" meant the "The Flowering of Youth" or the blossoming and hope of a nation and people. Remember, that at this time, Korea was divided into three kingdoms. It was the goal of the Hwarang to unite and defend Korea, a country that had been besieged by attackers for centuries. The Hwarang sought to capture and define the spirit of Korea and Koreans, thus maintaining their cultural integrity as a people.

The Hwarang spirit is perfectly embodied in the life and story of

Sadaham. Sadaham was only sixteen when he became a Hwarang and, due to his great skills, strong character, and pleasant appearance, he had many followers. When King Chinhung ordered an attack on a neighboring state, Sadaham wanted to join the ranks. At first the King refused because of Sadaham's youth, but Sadaham was determined to fight and he insisted. The King made him assistant general. When the battle began, Sadaham was the first to enter the gate of the city under siege. His attack was so formidable that his army annihilated his foe, and Sadaham became a great hero. For his service the King offered Sadaham a large reward of land and servants but Sadaham refused. He simply felt it his duty to be of service to his country and therefore did not need a reward.

The Buddhist monk and scholar, Won-Kwang, who lived during this time and was personal advisor to the King, formulated and wrote down the code of living for the Hwarang in his "Five Commandments."

The "Five Commandments" are:
1. Loyalty to the King and country
2. Filial piety to parents
3. Sincerity to friends
4. Non-retreat in battle
5. Selectivity in killing of another human being.

To a young man at the time, there was no greater honor than to be part of the Hwarang. It was reserved for only the youth of nobility.

As Korean history progressed, the order and code of the Hwarang spread throughout the country, eventually becoming available to the common man. Eventually, the great secrets found a public forum in the art of Taekwondo. The ten creeds of Taekwondo, then, stemmed directly from the "Five Commandments" of Won-Kwang.

The ten creeds of Taekwondo are:
1. Be loyal to your country.
2. Be obedient to your parents.
3. Be lovable between husband and wife.
4. Be cooperative between brothers.
5. Be respectful to your elders.
6. Be faithful between teacher and student.
7. Be faithful between friends.
8. Be just in killing.

9. Never retreat in battle.

10. Accompany decisions with action and finish what you start.

In my school, I teach these ten creeds to my students. They still remain the philosophical backbone of Taekwondo and are timeless in their value. The ten creeds became my own personal bible during my years in Seoul after the war.

Over the next six months, our numbers at the open-air theater grew steadily to about 50. As we became more organized in our group and training procedures, simultaneously, the university became more organized and was able to accept us as the official Martial Arts Club of Yonsei University. The university also provided us with an indoor space to train. I became president of the club. Immediately, we began to set up informal tournaments with different university clubs, and we always emerged the winner because our techniques were sharp and advanced. During these tournaments, I developed a particular style of fighting known as counter-attack. It was a style perfectly suited for me because I was not very big, but I was strong and quick.

The counter-attack style of fighting allowed me to gain an advantage over opponents. In employing counter-attack, I would initiate a particular move against my opponent only partially, not to strike and get points, but solely to instigate a response or move. Once my opponent responded with a specific move to counter my 'false' move, I would quickly locate an opening and strike him in the empty spot for points. This style is complex, demanding alertness and quick thinking, yet it is extremely powerful. I won numerous tournaments using counter-attacks. It is a particularly effective strategy when facing an opponent of equal strength or ability because to defeat such an opponent you must create an advantage. In using counter-attack, the opponent is beaten, in effect, by tactic as well as technique.

I had been in Seoul about a year participating in informal tournaments when the Moo Duk Kwan Institutes began to re-establish themselves and sponsor tournaments on an official level. These tournaments were held on both city and regional levels. Since almost all the martial arts activity in Korea at that time was centered in Seoul, there was little difference between the levels. I joined the tournaments as often as I could and, with relative ease, progressed to the higher levels. All the competitors were black belts; however, in those days, there was only one weight division. It was not unlikely that one would find himself facing a much larger opponent. Therefore, it was wise to know something about the opponent before you stepped out on the mat with him. Through a process of elimination, I could deduce who my prospective opponents were, and I surveyed them during their bouts carefully, not only to assess their ability but to carefully observe their fighting styles. Most martial artists relied on specific moves that were comfortable or well suited to them. My best move, for instance, was the hop sidekick because I was fast and very accurate with it. I spent a good deal of time at the tournaments watching others fight. I would size up my opponents and prepare a fighting strategy. Then, with my club members, I trained in that particular style.

A great martial art master once said: "In order to achieve victory you must place yourself in your opponent's skin. If you don't understand yourself, you will never win. If you understand yourself, you will win fifty percent of the time. If you understand yourself and your opponent, you will win one hundred percent of the time."

Applying this principle in one important tournament, I concluded that my first few matches on the regional level would be no problem if I fought up to my abilities. No major changes in my fighting style would be needed. The big match, however, would be the semi-final. My opponent in the semi-final match would most likely be a very strong fighter from a university in Pusan. He was well known and I had noticed him in earlier bouts. I decided to have a closer look at his technique. During his next match I watched him closely and took notes. Sitting high up in the gymnasium bleachers, I noted that his favorite kick was the sidekick. No one could attack him because his sidekick was so strong. It seemed to rip right through the block and score points. He won his matches easily. The only way to beat him, I thought, would be by speed and not strength.

Since the semi-final match was scheduled almost a week away, I had time to train. First, I drilled myself on the hop sidekick on my own, concentrating on the speed of execution. Then, I chose two members of my club who fought in a similar style to my opponent. We worked long and hard hours, sometimes pushing ourselves beyond our limits. I had my club members attack me with sidekicks while I responded with a hop sidekick at lightning speed. I also trained my eye to pick up the nuances of the sidekick so that I could detect the move almost before it began. After the week of training was completed, I felt ready and knew that I had a clear strategy.

If my opponent did his homework, as I am sure he did, he would expect to see the hop sidekick from me and the use of counter-attack. I would show it to him, yes, but with great speed and a little twist. I planned to execute the hop sidekick as soon as he started his move, not as my initial move. I simply wanted to antagonize him, make him feel that he could not execute a move without my quick response. If I gained the advantage in this way, the match would be mine.

Entering the gymnasium on the day of the semi-final match, I felt nervous but sure of myself. If I followed my plan, all would go well, I hoped. My techniques were well honed. But, techniques are not all. I had learned through years of experience that thinking plays a large part of being a martial artist. My mental state was also well honed. In a tournament setting, when conditions for a challenge are pre-set and a martial artist can display all that he has learned, tactics become equally as important as technique. The gym was filled with spectators and banners; cheers echoed throughout. However, all that existed in my mind was the mat, the stage upon which I was about to perform.

I stood off to the side, stretching and loosening my muscles and joints. The match would soon begin. I felt butterflies in my stomach. Then, I heard my opponent's and my name being called over the loudspeaker for the semi-final match. I stepped out onto the mat slowly and deliberately feeling both relaxed and wound up tight simultaneously.

My opponent stood facing me. Our gazes locked. He was a muscular fighter, larger than me, with fierce determination and concentration in his eyes. "Speed, speed," I whispered to myself. Beside this, my mind was blank; I was all impulse and perception.

Those first few seconds before the match begins is an important moment. In any competitive match, not to mention an actual life or death combat, the psychological battle begins even before the physical fighting has begun. The mind must be at perfect rest and non-anticipation; it must be free of all content and remain open, clear, yet focused. From this point of absolute zero, so to speak, you can defend and attack from any direction. Any sense of fear or agitation will disturb this readiness and, if your opponent is aware of it, victory is already theirs.

There is a classic story in the martial arts tradition that illustrates this point. It tells of a confrontation between a master of the Japanese tea ceremony and a rogue samurai. In a busy marketplace, the samurai bumped into the tea master's hip, and yet blamed the tea master for touching his sword. An argument ensued ending with the samurai threatening to kill the tea master. Gripped with fear, the tea master apologized profusely to the samurai.

This only whetted the samurai's appetite for further confrontation. He told the tea master that he must meet him in a field the next day with a sword and fight. The tea master would either die like a man in combat or be hunted down like an animal, the samurai said.

The tea master, beside himself with fear, didn't know what to do. So, he went to seek the advice of a local samurai warrior. After pleading with the samurai to help him, the samurai finally agreed to teach the tea master what he could in one day with the sword in order to defend himself. The tea master went out, bought a sword, and immediately began his instruction from the good samurai. Quickly, however, the samurai discovered that the tea master had no aptitude for the sword, and after a short period of time, the frustrated samurai gave up and told the tea master that his only recourse was to prepare himself to die the following day.

The tea master stood before the samurai in utter despair, already looking like a defeated animal. Then, because nothing else could be done, the samurai asked the tea master to prepare some tea for them. The tea master was surprised at this request, but conceded. The two men retired to the tea master's house where he prepared the tea in the perfect ritual that he had performed thousands of times. During this ritual the samurai noticed that the tea master's demeanor had suddenly changed from a broken, defeated man to a confident one with grace and power. Upon this observation, the samurai told the tea master that when he went to face the rogue samurai, act as if he were performing the tea ceremony. At first the tea master didn't understand. The samurai instructed him to clear his mind and be neither fearful of death nor desire life.

"Just hold your sword above your head with the awareness of the tea ceremony," the samurai said.

Then, the tea master understood.

The next day when the rogue samurai approached the tea master he noticed that the tea master had his sword raised and an expression of peace on his face. Expecting to see the tea master quivering in fear, the samurai began to feel uneasy. A few steps away, the samurai gazed into the eyes of the tea master and saw nothing but strength and confidence. Upon seeing this, the samurai's arms went limp and he turned away in defeat.

As the bell sounded for the start of my match in my semi-final round, we each took a step closer to the other, observing each other. Our movements were slow, precise, controlled. Both of us knew what to expect—or did we? My opponent stepped forward, apparently about to snap his leg in a sidekick to intimidate me. I leaped forward with a hop sidekick; it was so fast that I regained my position before he did. No points were exchanged. We were only testing each other. I had to resist initiating a move and just waited. He moved again, I responded again with a hop sidekick. This teasing continued a few more times, sometimes using my left foot, other times my right. He was confused and I saw that he was becoming flustered. He could not get near me without seeing a hop sidekick that was faster than he ever expected. My strategy seemed to be working.

When I thought it was appropriate, I moved closer to him. We were going for points now. I waited for his next move. It came and I approached as if to give another hop sidekick, but instead spun around with my back foot and hit him in the chest with a turning back kick. It had worked. I had scored first and, in doing so, utterly surprised him. I had the advantage. Quickly I seized the opportunity, found his 'mental' empty spot and scored again with a hop sidekick to his stomach area. It all happened so fast, 2 quick points with a surprise counter-move and a quick offensive move. The strategy had worked.

Two points down, my opponent was now flustered. I shifted my strategy again and went on the offensive, exploding with a series of kicks. None had scored. I felt his defenses weakening and I sensed he was expecting more counter-attack moves. He backed away to readjust himself and I stepped in with a jumping high sidekick to the face for the final point of the match. I had won 3 points to none, thanks to my strategy of counter-attack.

Three days later, I met an opponent in the finals. I went into the match with much confidence after winning a tough bout in the semi-final. This alone seemed to intimidate my new opponent. The match was somewhat anti-climactic. He was a fine martial artist, but his technique was not as refined or strong as the opponent in the semi-final. His weaknesses were more evident and I took advantage right away. The final match was a two-minute bout and I scored four points to his one, winning easily. My style was controlled with no surprises. I had become champion at 20 years old.

The trophy that I won that day has been on display in a trophy case at the Yonsei University gymnasium ever since the tournament. It is a tall trophy on columns, a gold-plated figure of a martial artist executing a sidekick. I am filled with memories whenever I think about it. I was so proud then to have won it because it symbolized my life and work in the past 10 years, and my life and work to come.

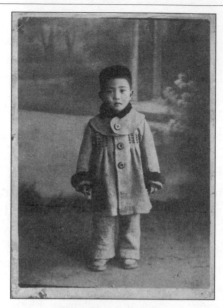

Richard Chun in childhood.

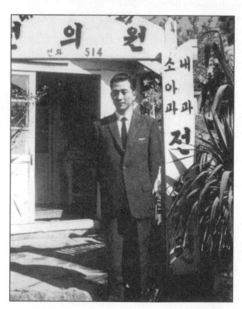

Richard Chun in his Junior Year at Yon Sei University. Photo taken in front of his father's hospital in Cheju Island after the Korean War, 1954.

CHAPTER 4

In the Lion's Den

After the Korean War, I lived in Seoul in a one-story house in Bukahyum-Dong village with my brothers and sister. The house was built in traditional Korean style that meant that it included an ondol bang. This unique feature of a Korean house was a family room with a hole built right into the floor. It went straight down to the earth below so that a fire could be made to warm the house and provide a gathering point for the family.

With my father and mother now living on Cheju Island and my eldest brother studying medicine in Japan, there were four of us in the house. One brother worked as a psychologist in a government office, the other was a student, and my sister was a diplomat in the Ministry of Foreign Affairs. I had recently joined them after a year of military service upon graduation from the university and was looking for a job. During the days, I read the "want ads" in the paper and went on interviews; not much to my liking came along. In the evenings, I gathered together with my brothers and sister around the fire to exchange the news and stories of the day.

"Soo Hong and Mae Kim are getting married," my sister told us one evening. "They met at a dance about six months ago. I'm happy for Soo Hong. Mae Kim is very pretty and well-educated," she added.

"We have to find someone for Rhin Moon, now that he's back and ready to begin his life," said my elder brother.

"Wait, wait," I said. "First I need to find a job."

"You may have to wait a long time then, Rhin Moon. Jobs are hard to come by these days. Everyone wants a good job," said my sister.

"Yes, maybe you could work at the docks, unloading and packaging fish," said my younger sister. Everyone laughed because they knew I disliked both the smell of fish and handling them.

One evening my elder brother said that he had heard from a friend who was a journalist about an opening for a sales position at Air France. This sounded good so we immediately contacted my brother's friend and found out that there were indeed two openings and that they were still accepting applications for a few more days.

"At the Bando Hotel," said my brother, speaking to his friend over the phone.

"The Bando Hotel," repeated my younger brother in an excited voice.

I also felt a sense of excitement rush to my stomach when I heard the name Bando Hotel. This hotel was the most luxurious in all of Seoul in the 1950's to the early 1960's. The finest companies had offices there, and even the President of Korea had a suite at the Bando Hotel. You could not even enter the hotel restaurant if you didn't possess American dollars or special coupons used only in the hotel.

"Are you going to apply?" said my sister.

"Yes," I replied. "I want this job."

The next morning I took a bus downtown. As I exited the bus across the street from the hotel, I looked up at it. The Bando Hotel took up an entire city block. It was the largest and most beautiful building in downtown Seoul, built during the construction boom after the war. It was modern, built of steel and glass. There was nothing else like it in Seoul. I was overwhelmed just looking at it, but when I entered the lobby for the first time, my mouth dropped in awe. A huge space with trees and a waterfall loomed before me. Throughout the lobby were plush chairs and sofas and large, exotic flower arrangements on coffee tables that perfumed the entire space. Soft colors created an effect of openness, and receptionists in maroon uniforms stood behind counters of deep teak wood.

I was escorted up to the second floor—the Air France offices—where I was immediately greeted by an attractive secretary.

Proudly, I announced that I was here to apply for the job opening. She led me over to a table where other candidates were already filling out application forms. When I finished, I was brusquely instructed to return in two days for a written examination.

"At 9:00 AM sharp," the secretary emphasized.

Two days later I arrived early and was brought to a large banquet room filled with long tables. The room looked like a gigantic classroom. The exam, sealed shut, had already been placed on the tables in front of each seat. There were hundreds of them. In the next half an hour people of all types—young and old, well dressed and casual-dressed, men and women—arrived and were promptly brought to their places. The test started as soon as we were given some simple instructions.

There was no way to prepare for such an exam. The questions were designed to test our attitudes about selling and salesmanship, about our present and future goals, about our work habits and patterns. We answered questions about hypothetical sales situations, and the test concluded with a short essay about our expectations of Air France and why we wanted to work for the company. It was the type of exam that upon finishing, one and a half hours later, you had no idea how you had performed.

As I walked out of the Bando Hotel that day with the hundreds of applicants, I noticed that many looked as if they had much more sales experience than I. My hopes were not very high. I was very surprised when I received a letter in the mail one week later, asking me to come for a personal interview. I had been chosen, out of those hundreds, to continue the evaluation process. I called immediately and scheduled an appointment..

On the morning of my appointment, I wore my best jacket and tie and stopped at the barbershop to get my hair trimmed. I felt confident and like a budding salesman as I entered the offices of Air France, but inside I was shaking like a brittle leaf. I announced my arrival to the secretary, the same one as before. Just her familiar presence put me at ease at bit.

"Oh, yes, Rhin Moon. You are here for the interview," she said. "Please have a seat. Mr. Kim will see you shortly."

Mr. Kim, I thought. He must be the boss. I wondered if he would be kind and what he looked like. I picked up a travel magazine on the coffee table and began to flip through it.

Soon, Mr. Kim appeared in the doorway of a room near the reception area. He was tall and young, well-dressed, with a very pleasant smile. I immediately felt comfortable with him.

"Rhin Moon, welcome to Air France. I am Mr. Kim. Congratulations on being chosen as a candidate for this position. Please come in," he said and gestured towards the open door.

As I entered the room, my nervousness, which had dissipated with Mr. Kim, suddenly hit me again like a blast of cold air. Seated around a large round table were four men, all older than Mr. Kim and all staring at me, stone-faced. I was introduced to each one and told to take a seat at the table.

The next thirty or forty minutes went by quickly. I remember hearing that 20 out of 200 candidates had been chosen for this round of interviews. I consciously tried to smile a lot and make eye contact, as my brother, the psychologist, suggested.

"Rhin Moon, why do you want to work for Air France?"

"Rhin Moon, are you prepared to work long and hard hours, sometimes with few results?"

"Rhin Moon, what would you do if ... "

"Rhin Moon, do you belong to any groups or associations where you could prospect for potential customers?"

"Rhin Moon, how long would it take ... "

"Rhin Moon ... Rhin Moon ... "

Finally, the interview was over and I left. I had no indication of how I had performed, yet I felt that I had done my best. I was satisfied with myself. One thing that I had learned during my years of training in the martial arts was that one must learn to overcome fears. This is the warrior spirit. The warrior must draw upon his or her inner strength to turn obstacles and fears into challenges and face these challenges head on, until you succeed. Most of the time you will find that your obstacles and fears are merely a figment of your imagination rather than being real. During that interview with all the executives of Air France, I felt my fear, but I recognized it as I had so many times on the mat during my training, and through strength and will power, I conquered my fear and did the best that I could.

The next few days however, were still spent in anticipation, waiting to hear if I had succeeded in the interview and would be accepted as a candidate. Every evening, the first thing my brothers and sister asked when they returned from their day at work or school was "did you hear anything yet?" They were supportive and comforting to me, even joking with me by asking if they would be able to get discounts on airfares when I got the job. They helped ease the tension during that time of waiting.

About a week after the interview, Mr. Kim called. He said that I had been one of six candidates chosen for a pre-appointment training for one week, after which two of us would be offered the job. He congratulated me and told me to report to the office on Monday of the following week. I dropped the phone after the call and cheered in excitement. My brothers and sister surrounded me and I told them the news. They all hugged and congratulated me, knowing that I didn't even get the job yet. But, we were happy that I had made it this far.

The week of training was demanding; we spent five full days together learning sales techniques, studying products, memorizing policies and procedures. We went through mock sales, learning how to overcome objections. For one week, we were absorbed in this world, six candidates, all after the same job, all intelligent and highly motivated, all getting to know each other, all leading to the final day where we had to complete a final test before the decision would be made. Only two of us would succeed. By the end of the week we all felt ready, yet none of us knew what to expect from the final test. Towards the end of our fifth day, Mr. Kim, our sales manager and instructor, made the announcement about the final test. We would be sent out to the field for an actual test sale to the public. The one twist was that our potential customer was to be chosen by our managers.

We were handed a typed paper with the name, position, address, and phone number of our potential client. One of us had to sell a ticket to a top model in the fashion industry, another to a government official, another a well-known soccer player. On my paper, it read: Mr. Chong In Hong, Chief Editor, Chosen Daily Newspaper.

My jaw dropped in surprise. My potential client was the chief editor of the most widely read newspaper in Seoul. My manager informed me that it was known that Mr. Hong was planning to attend a journalism conference in Paris next month. My job was to sell him a ticket to Paris on Air France.

That evening at home, seated around the fire with my brothers and sister, I told them about the final test and Mr. Hong. My sister said she had heard of him.

"He has the reputation of being a difficult man," she warned. "Our office sent a writer to work with him on an assignment. He is supposedly not easy to work with."

"This is going to be impossible," I said. "Thank you, sister," I added sarcastically.

The following morning I awoke with a sense of fear in my heart. In my mind I kept hearing my sister say "He is a difficult man," and my own voice in the background, weakly repeating, "This is going to be impossible." That morning, I was uncharacteristically slow in getting out of bed. I needed to reach deep down to find the motivation and tell myself that I have come this far already, only a little more to go. I would go see Mr. Hong, trust my instincts, overcome my fears, and simply do my best.

More than anything else our negative thoughts and feelings hold us back from achieving our goals in life. If we fill our minds with pictures and images of failing, then surely this will happen and we will say to ourselves, "I knew it." We must rid our minds of this negativity and instead, fill ourselves with the positive thought of "I can do it." Only then, are you calling forth all your reserves, making your chances that much better.

I walked slowly to his office that first morning, convincing myself that I had been properly trained. I was ready for anything. I saw the similarities between the task at hand and the martial arts. One overcomes fears through the knowledge that you have trained under the guidance of masters and that you have internalized your art. In the face of a great task, you must rise to the occasion and draw upon all that you have learned. I would attempt to do this, I convinced myself.

I entered the building of the daily newspaper around mid-morning. Many people were rushing in and out. On the lobby walls hung poster-size photographs that had once been published in the paper, along with blow-ups of historic front pages. Mr. Hong's office was on the second floor. I took the elevator and as the doors opened, I walked into a large reception room with a desk surrounded by plants. Along the wall was a row of chairs and a coffee table with copies of the daily newspaper on top. I approached the secretary, introduced myself, and asked if I may see Mr. Hong.

"Do you have an appointment?" she asked.

"No, I do not," I said.

"Mr. Hong is a very busy man," she said. "He usually doesn't see anyone without an appointment."

"Yes, I know, but maybe I could see him briefly between appointments," I said. The secretary arched her eyebrows in an inquisitive manner.

"And whom shall I say is calling, and with what purpose?" she asked.

"My name is Rhin Moon Chun and I am with Air France."

"I'll see what I can do," she said.

I sat on a chair along the wall and waited, and waited, and waited. All day in fact, I sat on that chair and watched people go in and out of his office. Occasionally he would emerge, have a brief chat with his secretary and then retreat back again into his office. Once, he glanced over to me, spoke briefly with his secretary, and disappeared again.

Mr. Hong was a large man with a close-cropped haircut and deep, bushy eyebrows; his forehead was furrowed with wrinkles and his eyes were penetrating. He looked quite imposing. He wore a plain blue suit with a blue and red striped tie. His hands were large and his shoes, shined to a bright polish, seemed to stick a long way out from under his pant legs. I tried to smile when he glanced over to me, but my mouth seemed frozen.

Throughout the day, I sat quietly, collecting myself, sometimes picking up the newspaper to read an article, mostly just observing the reception room and smiling at the secretary if she glanced my way. Just before the end of the day the secretary approached me and apologized. She said Mr. Hong would be unable to see me that day. Try tomorrow, she suggested.

The following morning I arrived in Mr. Hong's office at 8:30, a half hour before the business day began. My fear had diminished somewhat and been replaced by a headstrong determination to see him. When Mr. Hong arrived about 20 minutes later he noticed me. I smiled and nodded; he nodded back. His day began with numerous phone calls and appointments, and about mid-morning, he left the office, returning a little before lunch. The secretary suggested that I get something to eat, but I really didn't want to leave and miss an opportunity to see him. She told me that Mr. Hong always took a half-hour lunch at this time and would not be seeing anyone, so I quickly went down to the coffee shop in the main lobby, had a sandwich and I was back in Mr. Hong's reception room 20 minutes later.

An hour later, his secretary glanced over at me and said that Mr. Hong would see me now.

"You have been very patient," she said. "Good luck."

She opened the door to his office and announced my name to Mr. Hong. By now, I felt as if I were entering a sacred temple, off limits to all but a select few. Immediately, I was struck by the size of the office. I was expecting a large office with the most elegant furniture, but instead, Mr. Hong's office was a cramped space with a simple desk next to a window. On the desk sat a large typewriter, a couple of phones, and piles of newspapers, magazines, and books. The walls were bare except for a few photographs of himself with various personalities and more stacks of books and papers. In the corner was a small filing cabinet. He spoke first.

"You see that I'm a very busy man, yet you are patient and persistent. What can I do for you?"

I thought it best, since he obviously was a busy man, not to mince words.

"I am with Air France, sir," I said. "We have learned that you are about to travel to Paris for a conference next month. I would like to ask you to purchase your ticket from us."

"Yes, this is what I expected," he said. "My secretary told me you were from Air France."

"Yes, sir. Seeing that you are traveling to Paris, what better airline to chose than Air France. We will promise excellent service, of course."

"Oh, yes, yes, I'm sure of that," he commented. Then, he sat in silence for a while.

That's when I noticed his diploma on the shelf. The university he had attended was the archrival of mine, Yonsei University. It didn't make me feel good. In fact, it made me feel as if the task at hand would be that much harder to accomplish. I began to feel cramped in his little office. In Korea, we have an expression for this kind of situation. It is like being in a lion's den. A lion's den is a place where obviously you cannot relax making it difficult to achieve your goal. Trying to sell Mr. Hong an airline ticket in his office was like being in the lion's den. I would have to be at my best to achieve what I came here to accomplish. He interrupted my train of thought with his blunt response.

"I'm afraid that will be impossible," he said. "I appreciate your persistence in waiting to see me, but I cannot buy a ticket from you."

So this is it, I thought. Is it all over? Should I just thank him for seeing me, get up, and walk out disappointed? All that time, taking the test, being interviewed, going through the training for nothing. I couldn't let it slip away in one moment. I spoke.

"Do you have one already, sir?" I said.

I waited for his response, and to my surprise, he softened up a bit.

"No, no; it's nothing like that. There is another problem."

"Yes, sir," I said, trying to understand.

"You see, Mr. Chun ... I am on the board of directors of KTB. Do you know what KTB is?"

I sat expressionless, just listening.

"KTB is the Korean Travel Bureau. We are a government agency that arranges flights for dignitaries, government personnel, and public figures. I'm afraid I can't go against my own business. You see ... we are competitors," he said.

I was shocked, of course, to hear this. I did not know about KTB, and frankly, at this point, I felt that my chances of selling him a ticket were close to none. Yet, I thought it best not to reveal these feelings to him.

"Oh, yes sir, I know this," I replied without skipping a beat. "I just thought you might explore how Air France can service you. I can show you an itinerary."

Then, Mr. Hong leaned back in his chair and put his hands on his head. He might have been contemplating something or just getting bored or impatient with me. I couldn't tell which, but I had to say something or else I knew that I would lose the sale for good. I interrupted his train of thought.

"Mr. Hong, let me be honest with you. I am really a trainee with Air France, not actually hired; I was assigned to sell this ticket to you as part of a test sale. If I sell the ticket to you I will be hired."

Then, I looked into Mr. Hong's eyes trying to judge his response. Being honest with him at that moment came spontaneously, much like a kick or punch emerges quickly and naturally in a bout where you suddenly see a new opening. I did not know how he would respond, yet I tried it. After a while, he rolled forward in his chair and, to my surprise, said, "I can't promise you anything, but let me see an itinerary tomorrow morning."

"Yes, sir," I said bounding up from my seat. "Thank you."

"I am not promising anything, I said," he reminded me as I left his office.

I rushed back to Air France and told my manager that Mr. Hong would like to see an itinerary.

"An itinerary?" Mr. Kim asked. "Are you sure, Rhin Moon?"

"Yes, yes," I replied, as his eyes grew larger and larger, filled with disbelief.

The following morning I was the first to see Mr. Hong. Our meeting was brief. I showed him the itinerary. He looked it over carefully and said, "Rhin Moon, you are a determined young man and you are also honest. I like that. You have the makings of an excellent salesman. I have thought long and hard about this and I can't believe what I'm about to do, but I will buy my ticket from you. Congratulations."

I stood and bowed to Mr. Hong.

"Thank you, Mr. Hong, thank you," I said.

"Now, let's take care of this today so I don't have to worry about it," he instructed.

I ran back to the offices at the Bando Hotel and told Mr. Kim the news. He was completely shocked and admitted to me that he did not expect me to sell the ticket to Mr. Hong. In fact, he knew that Mr. Hong was a director of KTB. In an hour, the travel arrangements were completed, and by mid-afternoon, I had delivered the ticket to Mr. Hong's office.

Two days later, Air France hired me. I was the only candidate to sell a ticket to their potential customer in the test sale. The other candidate, who was hired even though he did not sell his ticket, soon became a top salesman at Air France. As for me, I quickly rose to district manager and took charge of the Kwang Ha Moon Branch. My career at Air France spanned a successful five years until I decided to move to America to further my education.

I will never forget my experience with Air France, particularly how I got the job. I attribute my success in selling the ticket to Mr. Hong to my life as a martial artist. Through my training in the martial arts, I had developed the qualities of patience and persistence. I also learned that I could not master all the techniques and forms right away. There are just too many. It required much time and patience, working on one skill at a time, carefully and diligently, until it became second nature. Gradually, I realized that with patience and persistence, I had transformed myself into a martial artist with hundreds of moves at my fingertips and, equally important, a philosophy and tradition deep within me.

These qualities—patience, persistence, quickness, honesty, integrity—were deeply ingrained in my being and behavior. Only my development as a martial artist could have prepared me for this.

Often in life you will be placed in situations where you must spontaneously draw upon your inner resources. Life will demand that you rise up above your everyday existence, overcome obstacles, and become something greater than you are. If you have not developed these inner resources and qualities, then when you are called to draw upon them, they will not be available to you. If you do have these qualities and they are part of your being, then success will be yours in any endeavor. This is what the tradition of the martial arts teaches, this is what it means to be a warrior, and this is what you create in your life.

Shortly after Air France hired me, my brothers and sister organized a celebration party at our home with some friends. It was a night filled with happiness, warmth, and comfort. We gathered around the ondol bang and told stories and danced and laughed. During the evening, I remember a moment when I was describing my experience in Mr. Hong's office to my family and friends. I said, "I had been in the lion's den and came out victorious."

CHAPTER 5

In America

Life suddenly became filled with unexpected journeys. I'm not talking about the free vacation to Tokyo in my second year with Air France, or the trip to Paris for a manager's conference. After five years at Air France, having risen to become sales manager, I now found myself on a plane headed for the United States. It was not a vacation or business trip. I was moving to America.

"I'm going to study business at George Washington University in Washington, D.C.," I told the elderly couple who sat next to me on the flight. They were traveling to the U.S. to visit their son who practiced law in Washington.

"Why study in America?" the elderly man asked. "Why leave Korea?"

"What was your job in Seoul?" the elderly woman asked.

These questions triggered off a conversation with this couple that lasted, intermittently, throughout the entire flight.

"In Seoul, I worked as a sales manager for Air France," I said.

Their eyes lit up in surprise. They knew that I was leaving a very good job at a time when good jobs were hard to find. They didn't have to ask the next question. I saw it in their faces.

"Yes, it was a good job and I earned good money," I said. "And I lived the high life, too—meeting interesting people, dining and dancing in the fanciest restaurants and nightclubs, free vacations every year."

"Then why leave all that, and Korea?" asked the elderly man.

"And your family," added the elderly woman.

They were a sweet couple. The woman had a round face with a small nose. He was short and stocky, handsome, with a dark hue to his skin. These were good questions they were asking me.

"One day after work, I was walking home alone and suddenly I began thinking about my future, you know, my destiny. I asked myself—Where would I be in 5 or 10 years?"

"Did an answer come?" said the elderly man.

"Yes," I said. "And I didn't like it. The answer was ... in the same spot."

The elderly couple looked puzzled.

"Being Korean," I explained to them, "and working for a foreign company, there was no opportunity for me to really advance. The highest I could go was to become a sales manager. And I had already accomplished that."

I looked into their faces for understanding, and also, for approval. I continued telling my story.

"I wanted more in life. So, I began to think of what other skills and experience I had besides sales, and there were none really. It is true that I am a black belt in Taekwondo and I continue to train. It is a very important part of my life," I said. "Maybe, I will use that someday."

I didn't realize, then, that those words would prove to be so prophetic.

The elderly couple seemed to understand my plight and they were impressed when I told them I was a martial artist.

"One of the many things that I have gained from the martial arts, of which I am very grateful for, is the inner strength to make changes when changes become necessary in my life. If I feel fear and uncertainty facing something new, I know that by facing these fears and uncertainties and working hard to overcome them, that I will achieve my desires and, ultimately, become the person I was meant to be. I believe in this. It has happened to me many times in the training hall during my practice facing an opponent or working on perfecting a move or performing a difficult breaking technique."

They nodded in understanding. I continued.

"I knew that I had to leave Air France. It was a hard decision and I faced many fears, but I had to do it. That's when I decided to get a degree in business."

"You are a very brave and wise young man," said the elderly woman.

"Yes, but you still haven't explained to us why you choose to study in America, " said the elderly man.

"In America," I explained, "they are teaching the most advanced theories in business and marketing and I want to take advantage of the opportunity to study there. I feel I can get these skills in America very quickly and then go back to Korea to work. My aunt lives in Washington with her husband and family and they have invited me to stay in her home while I'm studying there."

During my conversation with the elderly couple, I discovered that he was a retired government official and his wife was a schoolteacher. After the war their son went to study in America and stayed. Talking to them helped to make my trip to America easier for me simply by their presence. They eased any lingering anxiety I had about leaving Korea and coming to America, which was a big step out into the unknown for me. Just hearing about their son, who was so successful in America, seeing their interest in me, which was so simple and sincere, and verbalizing my story, which helped me realize my fears were really illusion anyway, I felt better. I had told them my full story, except for one detail.

It was true that I left a good job at Air France, where I was making good money, however, the one detail that I left out of my story was that I was coming to America with only $200.00 in my pocket, and not much more to my name. The reason for my financial state, then, was that about a year before I left Air France, a friend asked me if he could borrow a large sum of money from me for a "good investment," he said. When I asked him to start paying me back, he informed me that the investment went bad and that he was bankrupt. I had lost my money. What was left in my savings would be sent over to me by my brother, but only in small increments because at that time Korean citizens were not allowed to bring out more than 200 hundred dollars in U.S. currency from the country.

As I handed my bankbook over to him at a family gathering to wish me good luck and good-bye, he told me to be careful. The farewell party was a warm and tearful event. My family was supportive of my decision and all said they would miss me dearly. My parents, however, were not present because my father's busy practice on Cheju Island prevented him from leaving. The elderly couple on the flight reminded me of my parents in many ways and substituted for their presence.

When I arrived in Washington, my aunt and uncle with two of their children met me at the airport. On the drive back to Washington, they asked me all about my plans and said how happy they were to see me. By evening, I was set up in comfortable room in their home in suburban D.C.

I spent the next few weeks getting to know the city and my new family. Washington surprised me. It was a clean city with many grand buildings, but having just come from Seoul, bustling and teeming with people, Washington actually seemed like a rural town to me. The downtown area was small and the suburbs seemed almost quiet and empty. My aunt had four children, but two were away at college in California, which opened up a room for me. Within a few weeks of arriving in Washington, I began a Master Degree in

Business and Marketing at George Washington University.

Classes were good and I enjoyed studying. I also began to make new friends and enjoyed doing things with them. Not wanting to be a financial burden on my aunt and uncle, I soon wanted to find a job to help me pay some living and entertainment expenses. About a month after I enrolled at the university, a Korean friend whom I met in one of my classes found a job for me as a waiter in a Chinese restaurant. So, in a little more than a month after arriving in D.C., I was going to school, had a home, and a job. I would say that I was getting off to a good start in America. However, my perfect life didn't last very long.

It soon became obvious to me that the job at the restaurant was not working out. It wasn't so much that I couldn't remember the names of the drinks and how to make them or even the fact that I couldn't get used to accepting tips and that I would often give them back to the customers, but it was the idea that I was a waiter. Frankly, I felt ashamed about it. In Korea, working for Air France, my circle of acquaintances was from a very high level, including government officials and business leaders. On numerous occasions at the restaurant, I ran into these same people whom I knew from my days at Air France. It made me feel uncomfortable and I quit after about six weeks of work.

As events lead to other events, after about five months in D.C. with one semester at George Washington University behind me, I found myself again on an unexpected journey, this time on a bus heading for New York with the help wanted ads from the New York Times on my lap. A friend had told me that there were many more opportunities in New York and that he was sure I would find something.

"Don't worry about a place to stay," he said. "I have friends there who will let you stay with them for a while."

The bus ride to New York was a bit depressing. Had I failed my relatives in Washington? Had I failed myself? The last month had been a tough one. I began to feel frustrated with myself. I wanted to focus on my studies, but also needed to find work to finance my expenses at school. After I left the restaurant job, I immediately began looking for more fulfilling work. About a month later, I was hired by Air Canada in their sales force; I was back in the airline business, not really what I wanted or expected. It was a good job, but didn't pay well and it demanded much of my time, which cut into my studies. I soon began to feel that I was losing my purpose and focus for being in America, which was to study. After completing my first semester at the university, I was faced with an impossible decision—leave school for a semester while I work or stay in school and quit my job at Air Canada. Both choices were not what I wanted. So, for some time I was torn between these two opposites, in a dilemma of which I saw no solution.

Here, again, my training in the martial arts helped me. I knew that when you set a goal, you must be determined to achieve that goal no matter what obstacle presents itself. It is very important to stick to your goal and never give up. I was caught between two choices that were not satisfactory to me until a friend suggested I try New York where I may be able to accomplish both. How? I didn't know, but I was willing to try. So, one day, I boarded a bus and decided to take my chances.

When I stepped out of the bus station onto the streets of New York, I finally felt that I entered the United States I had imagined. The crowds, noise, and excitement of the city were much greater than even Seoul, and everything, was on such a grand scale, so large. I felt exhilarated, and at the same time, horrified.

With the New York Times in my hand, I thumbed through the want ads checking off any job that looked appealing. I paid particularly close attention to the location of the jobs to see if I could get an interview right away. I saw job openings of all sorts: waiters (no thanks), store managers (not bad), teachers (couldn't do that). Then, I saw an ad for Fairchild's Publications as a bookkeeper and accountant, no experience necessary, and the location was just a few blocks away. I called and asked if I could stop in for an interview.

"How about 10 minutes from now? I just happen to be close by," I said.

Only an hour in New York and I had my first interview. Maybe my luck was changing. Maybe my friend was right. There seemed to be unlimited opportunities in New York.

I walked into the office of Fairchild's Publications ten minutes later. The Director of Employment, a pleasant man in a striped tie greeted me. We sat and began to talk. He asked me questions about myself and why I was in the U.S. Then, he began to talk about himself. I soon discovered that he was a veteran of the Korean War and had a strong liking for Koreans. He told me about his experience during the war, and about Fairchild's Publications.

Fairchild's was a large publishing house specializing in trade newspapers and journals. They were looking for young man who was interested in learning bookkeeping and accounting. Training would be on the job. I was excited to hear this because I wanted to study business anyway.

"I will work very hard, sir," I said.

"Of course, " the director said.

To my surprise and overwhelming joy, I was hired right then and there. I would start in one week to give me enough time to move from Washington. I returned to Washington and told my aunt about the unexpected news. She was shocked.

"You're moving where?" she asked me when I told her that I would be leaving in a few days. "Where will you stay?"

"My friend said I could rent a room with a Korean friend he knows there," I said.

Of course, she tried to persuade me to stay in Washington and expressed her worry and concern about my moving "to that big and unfriendly city." I had already made up my mind by then and told her not to worry.

"I can take care of myself, auntie," I said and promised to call and visit often.

In a couple of days, I was situated in a small room in a small apartment on 72nd Street and Broadway. I began work a few days later.

My English had improved dramatically since being in the U.S., but not until the job at Fairchild's did I encounter and learn American slang. I was the only foreigner in the office and my co-workers took particular delight in teaching me expressions such as 'hit the road, Jack,' or 'off to the funny farm.' They found it hilarious when I used these expressions in conversation. The job, itself, was excellent; I learned a lot about business and my co-workers were good people who treated me with respect and friendship.

As soon as I arrived in New York, I applied to a number of universities. I was accepted in all, but only Long Island University in downtown Brooklyn offered me a scholarship. I was also able to get some financing through the Korean-American Foundation to get my MBA in Marketing. I immediately enrolled in night classes.

Soon, I moved to Brooklyn, closer to the campus, and went to university a few nights a week while working during the day. Life was very full. The weeks went by with great speed, and I felt that there was not enough time in the day to accomplish all that I wanted to do, juggling work and study.

When the weekend came, I enjoyed meeting other foreign students at the Foreign Student Organization on campus, and occasionally visited my aunt and uncle in Washington. With my new friends in New York, we often went out to restaurants, parties and even dancing. It was through this connection that I met three other Korean black belts who were also studying at the university: Master Cho, Master Lee, and Master Shin. Soon, we all became friends and did many things together.

For some reason, of which I'm still not quite sure, I didn't bring my doboks to America with me. Maybe I figured that I was coming here temporarily only to earn a degree and then return to Korea. I had no intention of training seriously or teaching in the U.S. Yet, it soon became obvious that life had other plans for me, and in a couple of months I found myself on the subway three times a week, headed for Sigward's Sports Academy to teach Taekwondo to westerners.

Sigward's was located in midtown Manhattan and it was one of the first public health clubs to open in New York City. Mr. Sigward, a gentle and warm man in his late fifties, had opened the academy ten years earlier and offered weight training, boxing, calisthenics, basketball, and now Taekwondo. Mr. Sigward had a lifelong interest in fitness, worked out regularly and seemed to be in excellent shape, but mainly he was an astute businessman. The sports academy was very successful and Mr. Sigward was very rich. In many ways he was ahead of his time with regards to how he ran his health club.

On a Sunday outing a month before I started with Sigward's, I casually mentioned to Master Lee that I missed practicing and teaching martial arts. There was no competition among us, and Master Lee suggested that I visit Sigward's. A few days later I was sitting across the desk of Mr. Sigward, a large man, for an interview.

"You're 28 years old, Master Chun," said Mr. Sigward.

"That's right, sir," I said, feeling a bit intimidated by his presence. He had such big hands, I noticed.

"And you want to teach Taekwondo here?" he said.

"That's right, sir," I said. He played with a glass paperweight as we talked, sometimes looking into it as if it were a crystal ball.

"I think it's a good idea," he said, pausing for a second. Then, he added, "What is Taekwondo?"

I almost laughed.

"Let me show you," I said.

I stood up and went through some simple hand movements while Mr. Sigward watched. He stopped me midway through.

"Good, good. That's very good," he said. "I'll announce this to the members and we'll see how many are interested."

A month later, I started classes with ten students, training them in a small, dusty room covered with hard canvas mats. They were young men in their twenties, who worked in offices, stores, or went to school. Mostly, they were intrigued with the mystery of Asian fighting techniques, and interested in the philosophy of the martial arts. They were full of questions about the Taekwondo tradition and myself. During the workout, they were very physical, and sparring was their favorite part of training. Because of this, I was very physical with them, training them roughly. These handful of students were my first in the U.S. Eventually, they would all become my friends and many would go on to earn their black belts, some opening up schools of their own in different parts of the country.

I continued in this routine for nine months—working, studying, and now teaching martial arts—until an unfortunate incident took place that changed everything. Mr. Sigward died suddenly in his sleep of a heart attack. Apparently he was in good shape, but looking back from today's perspective of health and fitness, his diet was not very good, being too high in fatty foods. I felt a great loss upon Mr. Sigward's passing. He was a man of dignity and vision from whom there was much to learn from. He also gave me my first opportunity to teach martial arts in the America. I am forever indebted to him for that.

Even with the loss of Mr. Sigward, the sports academy continued to function; however, it was a time of big change for the academy and I felt that I could no longer rely on it. I continued teaching there, but began to look around for other places to teach. I also recognized at this time my desire to have my own martial arts school, but I was unclear about how to make that dream a reality. For about a year that desire lay still like a dormant seed. Until I met Dr. Kim.

At an alumni picnic for Korean students of Yonsei University, I was introduced to an elegant young man who I was informed worked as a Minister at the Korean Embassy. Dr. Kim had graduated Yonsei four years earlier than I. Immediately, we hit it off as friends; we talked about Korea, our work, Taekwondo. It became clear from our very first meeting that we were destined to meet. After the picnic we saw each other often, and Dr. Kim who often hosted parties at his apartment always invited me to attend. It was at these parties that he showed his guests his many talents.

At a certain point during the party, he would announce that he was going to play the piano. The room always became hushed. Dr. Kim would approach the piano and take his seat on the piano stool. He was an elegant, handsome man with his hair neatly trimmed and combed, his face square and strong, exuding a sense of confidence and strength. He played classical music exquisitely.

"He almost became a concert performer," someone whispered in my ear as I listened to his first performance, "but foreign affairs was more interesting to him."

After the performances, as a change of pace, sometimes Dr. Kim would entertain us by demonstrating a few breaking techniques that he picked up from his study of Taekwondo. Everyone enjoyed his sparkling personality.

Thus began my lifelong friendship with Dr. Kim. We saw each other frequently, attending parties, going out to eat at restaurants, seeing friends. Soon after meeting him, perhaps the second or third time we saw each other, he asked me what my long-range dreams and desires are.

"I've been thinking a lot about owning my own school for the martial arts, but I am not sure exactly how I will accomplish this. I mean I'm still in school and working..." I said.

Even before I finished I could see the excitement on Dr. Kim's face. We talked about it seriously for a while and a few days later, on his own, Dr. Kim offered to finance the start-up costs.

"Begin searching for a good location," he said.

Those words changed my life forever. Several months later, I opened the doors to my own school for the first time.

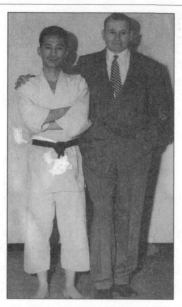

With Mr. Sigward of Sigward Sports Academy, New York City, 1962.

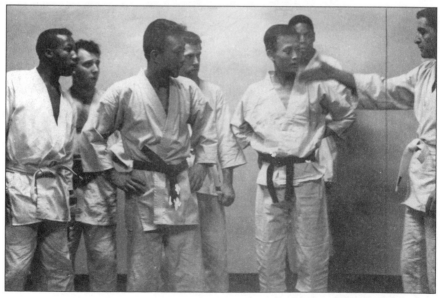

At Sigward Sports Academy, Richard Chun (center); Grandmaster Hyun Ok Shin (right), 1963.

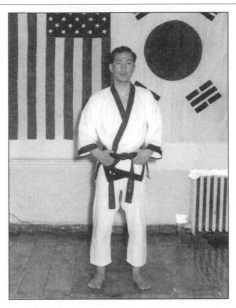

At the first school of Richard Chun Taekwondo Center, New York City, 1964.

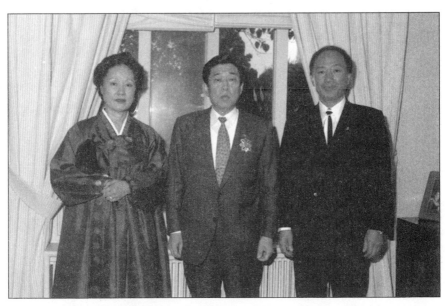

At award ceremony, Dr. Un Yong Kim, president of World Taekwondo Federation & I. O. C. member; Mrs. Un Yong Kim (left); Richard Chun (right).

CHAPTER 6

My Own School

Advancing through the ranks of a new color belt is the outer sign of progress and mastery for the student in the art of Taekwondo. This advancement requires hard work and discipline. A specific number of hours in training and the precise knowledge of a required number of forms must be fulfilled. The physical challenge for the student is very demanding, and as a young master in my own school, I felt this challenge to be as much mine as theirs.

At the opening of my school in 1964, I had about twenty-five students, a few of whom had followed me from Sigward's Academy. They were mostly high school and college students who were serious about of the martial arts. As their teacher, I worked them hard, holding them to the same standards that I held myself to. In order to train them properly, I had to train hard myself. I often stayed late after an evening's practice session, till midnight or one o'clock in the morning, to prepare for the next day's class.

I felt this preparation was absolutely necessary. I now had my own school, my own students, and I wanted nothing less than complete success in my new business. During this time as a young master, I began to feel a deep responsibility for the development of my students and the seriousness of my art. I realized that I was in the process of achieving my goal of becoming a leader and a teacher of others. This role pleased and fulfilled me, and the first thing I learned was that when one desires to better others, you spontaneously better yourself, and in bettering yourself, you better others. There is a well-known saying that the teacher learns more than the student. There is deep truth in this. The flow of knowledge and learning, the give and take back and forth, was immediately apparent.

The tradition of the martial arts throughout time has always been intimately tied to leadership and teaching. As human beings, we are all together on the same journey in life. This journey leads us in the direction of growth towards increased happiness, discovering our potential, and a life of fulfillment. My way has always been through the martial arts, and if anyone decided to join me on that path, I would happily accept them as a student and work as hard for them as I would work for myself. The truth is that there is no difference between myself and my students, and the relationships that develop between master and student are often deep, touching, and long-lasting.

One relationship, in particular, during my early years as a master, comes to mind. Frank Fuentes, Jr. was one of my senior and best students at Sigward's. While still in high school he progressed to 1st Dan Black Belt. I believe he was my first student to advance to this level. He had lightning speed and could break boards hanging by a rope suspended 6 feet above the ground. I trained him with love and dedication and saw that he tried to learn everything he could from me. He was like a sponge soaking up the art of the martial artist. I grew to feel for him not only as his teacher, but also as his friend and brother. Upon his high school graduation, however, he decided not to follow me from Sigward's to my own school, but instead enlisted in the Army and volunteered to serve in Vietnam. I hated to see him go, yet wished him well in his choice. I heard from Frank a few times through letters from Vietnam, yet tragically he was killed six months later by a land mine. After I heard the news through Frank's parents, I continued to maintain a relationship with them for a while. Occasionally, I visited them at their home on Long Island and once I received a holiday card from them with the greeting "Dear Son ... from Mom and Pop." The card brought tears to my eyes.

I will never forget Frank and his parents. They have since retired to Texas and we maintain correspondence once or twice a year. I will always remember them as an integral part of my life and development as a teacher of the martial arts. I was sorry that he could not be part of my own school. He would have been a great asset, and who knows how far he would have gone as a martial artist. In his short life, he went far as a human being.

Three months after the school's opening, I held our first promotional test. I felt the students were ready. They demonstrated various forms and performed breaking techniques, striving for smooth and precise execution. I was very pleased with the results. Twenty students had passed, earning their new belts. We also had our first black belt, earned by a Columbia University student majoring in physics, who had great strength and speed. It was a major milestone for all the students and the school, so I decided to organize a celebration to officially announce the school's opening to coincide with their promotion. Of course, everyone was excited about this idea. After practice one evening, we decorated the school with streamers and banners and worked on a demonstration of kicks and punches. The students invited their parents and friends; I invited local business owners; Dr. Kim, my friend and advisor for the school, invited foreign dignitaries from the UN. He also agreed to preside over the celebration.

On the night of the celebration, I arrived early to do some last minute preparations. I remember the feeling of happiness and fulfillment that I had as I opened the doors to the school that evening. The reality of the school suddenly sunk in. I could not believe that I had my own school. It was mine, with my name attached. It seemed a miracle that I had come this far. Everything had happened so quickly since my arrival in the United States. I had left my job at Fairchild's to work as a marketing research consultant for IBM during the day and I was an owner of my own business, a school for the martial arts. Life couldn't have been fuller, and I was busier than I could possibly imagine. It was so exciting to see my dreams taking shape. During these days time passed by so quickly. I could only hope that success would continue.

The school was open three nights a week and on Saturdays. When we were open, I would rush uptown from my job at IBM on East 42nd Street and hurry to open the doors to see my students enter. I felt so proud of them. They would enter and bow to me, some saying the traditional Korean greeting, "Annyung Hashipnika Kwanjangnim Chun," and I would respond, "Hello, Mark," or "Welcome, Doug," along with a warm smile. On the night of the celebration, after completing a few final preparations, the school seemed alive as it never had been before. I went into the office to relax and waited for everyone to arrive.

The school, located on the second floor of a small building on First Avenue between 77th and 78th Street, was modest—a single wooden floor with floor to ceiling windows in the front and back and a mirror on a side wall. I placed photos of myself in various kicking positions on the wall as well as the American and Korean flag alongside the Moo Duk Kwan emblem. An office was situated in the front corner of the school and looked down onto the street below. I could see people as they walked by, and if they glanced up they would spot the banner that read "Richard Chun's Martial Arts School" that hung in the front window.

Soon, the students and guests began to arrive for the celebration. After some introductions and refreshments, the festivities began. Dr. Kim spoke eloquently about the tradition of Taekwondo, emphasizing the discipline needed for training in the martial arts. Then he introduced me. I thanked all the students for their hard work and dedication, and gave honor and recognition to the students who had advanced to a new rank. I wanted to keep the evening simple and move on to the demonstration, but unexpectedly, Dr. Kim rose again and approached me. He first bowed to me and then turned to face the audience.

"We want to give special honor tonight to Richard Chun, Master in the art of Taekwondo," he said. "Master Chun's vision to bring this martial art, the pride of Korean culture, to the U.S. is being realized in his school today. We wish him many years of success."

Everyone stood and clapped and cheered, and I was at a loss for words. I was deeply touched and honored by Dr. Kim's words, but I remember also feeling somewhat overwhelmed. I was only 29 years old, only two years in America, my English still improving. Yes, it was true that I was a Master of Taekwondo, but as a teacher and businessman, I was only a novice, only a white belt. Would I succeed in this endeavor here in the U.S.? Where would all this lead? And what experiences would come to me through my commitment to the martial arts? I could not answer these questions at this time, yet I knew that throughout my life, I never lacked the self-confidence and strong will to make my dreams come true. At times I had failed, been knocked over, or had lost, but I always got back up again with firmer and stronger conviction. This desire to overcome failures and limitations, to venture out into the unknown to discover and make something of oneself, is the essence of the Taekwondo tradition. It was so much a part of me now that it was me.

"Dr. Kim, thank you. Your words are truly inspiring to me," was all I could say.

The celebration continued with a demonstration of kicks and punches by the advanced students, then by myself. The sounds of 'ki-up,' the vocal release of energy and force in Taekwondo, resounded through the gym. The guests, sitting cross legged around us and standing along the walls, watched silently in awe.

After the celebration ended, Dr. Kim and I stayed late and talked about the evening. At one point during our conversation, he summed it up by saying, "tonight was the birth of the school." His words rang true, and soon afterwards, he became one of its children. Dr. Kim picked up his training again with me at my school.

In the weeks following the celebration, our numbers grew. We gained some new students, and I continued to train them all rigorously, discovering new areas where work was needed.

"More speed," I announced in a voice that carried over the sounds of students working out. "Quicker, quicker—this move must be done with speed."

For a few days, we had been working on the sidekick and I had noticed that except for a few advanced students, the majority were not mastering this form. I had been drilling them in the correct execution of the kick—knee up, pivot on the left foot, lean back, and snap the leg. Their technique was correct, yet the speed of the form was off; it was too slow. I also noticed that during the workouts many of the students tired easily, breathing heavily throughout the practice.

"Take five," I said and the students either sat on the gym floor or went off to drink some water. A few minutes later we all gathered together again. I had one of my best students demonstrate the sidekick with perfect execution.

"Notice how fast the leg snaps," I pointed out. "The power of this kick comes from speed. In fact, the power of all kicks comes from speed. Remember this: power is the result of correct technique plus speed. It will develop with constant practice."

The students returned to their drill but something was still lacking. What was it, I wondered. Soon, the answer dawned on me. My students needed to be more flexible and in better physical condition; a lack of flexibility and conditioning was slowing them down. I decided then that I would put more emphasis on this in the next few weeks. So I made some changes.

The following workout started off as usual. Two of my top students, Joe Hayes and Hector Eugui, Jr., who had been with me since Sigward's, led the group in a 20-minute warm-up of calisthenics and stretching. After the warm-up, our normal routine would be to break up into groups, based on rank, and practice the forms under my supervision. Today however, I came out from my office after the warm-up and instructed the students to continue. They were surprised, of course, but continued—for another twenty minutes. Then I had the entire group do short wind sprints across the gym floor. They did this for another 20 minutes, took a 3 minute break, and then we concluded the workout with half an hour of weight training and practice hitting the punch board. As the students left the gym that evening I overheard some grumbling and complaining under their breaths, but I said nothing. Instead, I continued with this training for a couple of weeks, putting in a little time to practice forms so they wouldn't forget. Soon, I began to notice results.

However, the students by now were close to a mutiny. I waited to see if anything would happen.

This change in routine is not unfamiliar in the tradition of Taekwondo. If the master sees some need for instruction, he fulfills that need. For instance, I remember during my student days in Korea our master would suddenly tell us to go to a nearby park and jog for a few hours. Occasionally, on a Saturday or Sunday, he would instruct us to go into the mountains outside of Seoul to practice in the presence of nature. I remember once we went to a river with a waterfall and did our calisthenics under the force of the water's powerful flow. There, in a small training hall in New York City, it was less exotic, but the principle was the same.

Finally, however, the students could no longer hold in their frustration and questioning. During a short break in a workout, one evening, one of my older students spoke up.

"Master Chun," he said respectfully, with a quick bow, "many of the students are asking why our practice sessions have changed. They have asked me to ask you." All the students stood attentively with eyes and ears open.

"Yes, it is time that I told you, although you probably can guess. It is not to create a mutiny among you, I assure you of that." Everyone laughed and felt a bit more at ease.

"I want to improve your physical condition," I said. "Without proper conditioning and flexibility, you cannot master the techniques. I saw a need for this some weeks ago."

The students bowed and understood, and from that day on we found the perfect balance between physical training and practice of techniques. I became very pleased with everyone's progress and soon decided that my students were ready to test themselves in local weekly tournaments, sponsored by the martial art schools in the area.

The next few months proved to be very exciting and rewarding. More students enrolled, and thanks to a contact made at the celebration, I was able to get some free publicity. A short article on the martial arts with my school mentioned appeared in the New York Post, and from this, an invitation to be interviewed on local TV.

The Joe Franklin Show was a late-night talk show televised on New York stations. I wasn't sure how much publicity I would get since the show aired late at night. Still, I was happy to appear. I arrived at the studio at 10:30 PM for a live taping at 11:00. When I met Joe, his warmth put me at ease since I still felt a bit uncomfortable with my English skills, particularly on television. He was a short, cheerful man and very intelligent in his questioning. He also seemed genuinely interested in the martial arts.

Dressed in my doboks, I sat and answered questions, a bit stiffly at first, about Taekwondo and the growth of the martial arts in the U.S. Joe made a joke about my bare feet and then asked me to demonstrate a few moves. I went over to an open area on the set and performed some advanced kicking techniques. Every time I yelled out "ya" the audience burst out in cheers. I laughed out loud. Then, Joe came over dressed in his suit and wanted me to instruct him in some kicking techniques. I demonstrated and Joe followed my lead. Whenever he performed a move, the audience clapped loudly. Finally, I presented him with an honorary black belt. It was a good experience and thanks to the show, a few students decided to join the school.

In six months, we had grown to over 45 students. Everyone was working hard. My best students were doing well at the Sunday tournaments. We were coming home with trophies that I began to display in the front window of the school for all to see.

Around this time, another incident occurred that further expanded and deepened my teaching ability. Six or seven months after the school opened, we held our second promotional test. Many students advanced, but not all. A few days later, two students entered my office after practice one evening. They had been training for about four months. They were average students, who worked hard and attended most practice sessions. One boy was small with red, bushy hair and the other one thin with light hair and very quick movements.

"Master Chun, " said the small one, "may we see you?" They stood at attention, quite stiffly, behind the chairs opposite the desk where I was sitting.

"Of course. Please sit down," I said. They did not. I noticed the seriousness in their tone. "What's on your mind?"

"Master Chun," said the small boy, "we weren't promoted to yellow belt and we have been training for four months."

"Don't we deserve it?" said the other boy.

I sat back and listened to them explain how they had worked hard and paid money for their training, and therefore felt that they should have earned their yellow belt. They spoke as if they had been holding a lot inside and were now letting it all out.

I was silent for a while and when I responded I spoke carefully and deliberately.

"I am very proud of the hard work both of you have put into your martial arts training," I said, "but I must tell you that a student doesn't advance just because of hard work. You must master the routines and train the required number of hours."

They both sat in silence, stone-faced, listening to my words.

"Both of you did not fully meet the requirements. That does not mean you are not making progress or that you are not good students. In a few months we will have another promotional test. I'm sure you will succeed then. Be patient and continue your hard work."

They seemed satisfied with my explanation, bowed, and left. Afterwards, I thought much about this incident and realized that they had fallen prey to a common misconception about training in the martial arts. They expected too much, just by virtue of being students in the school. This was not the correct attitude for a martial artist to have. They would need to meet the requirements for advancement, and not expect it just because they were simply present and paying for their lessons. I was disturbed by this incident, but realized that I must be partially to blame. I had been demanding much from my students in their physical training, yet now I saw that I needed to place more emphasis on their mental attitude. The growth of my school also meant the growth of myself as a teacher. Of this, I was very aware. Unfortunately, a few days later, the small, red haired boy dropped out of training, but the thin boy continued and developed into a fine martial artist. Since that evening with the two boys, however, I made another necessary change in my teaching technique.

In the tradition of Taekwondo, mental training must go hand in hand with physical development. Initially, it is taught orally—explaining to students about the qualities of respect, humility, patience, self-control. However, these mental attitudes are only words unless they are constantly reinforced through physical training. I began to spend more time with the students talking about principles of mental development and paid deep attention to see that these principles permeated their behavior and the atmosphere of the school.

Of course, some were part of our routine already. We showed respect by bowing to the teacher and other students before and after training and sparring. The students were already responsible for the cleanliness of the school to develop humility. I had divided them into small groups to stay late or arrive early to clean the gym like the tradition during my early years. I took every opportunity to include a point of mental development during practice.

One day, some students were working on their round kick, a difficult technique because it demands perfect balance. One student in particular was having trouble with the kick, and after numerous attempts, he became frustrated. He was getting angry with himself, stamping his foot on the gym floor and cursing himself under his breath. With each kick his frustration increased, and of course, his performance worsened. I interrupted the practice, and spoke to him for all to hear.

"You are working with a difficult kick," I said, "which will take time to perfect."

Then, looking to all the students I said, "Be patient with yourself when you train in the martial arts. Certain techniques will naturally come easier to you than others. Concentrate on what you must do and be patient. If you feel yourself becoming frustrated or angry, this will only slow your progress. Instead, have self-control and believe that with time and practice you will perfect the form."

The student, who was having difficulty with the round kick, continued his practice along with the other students. I began to teach these moral and mental aspects of the martial arts through these little incidents more and more. I wanted to teach self-control to avoid anger if a student was accidentally hit during a sparring match, or instill a willingness to try if a student could do only 30 push-ups instead of 50. It made a profound change in the quality of the school.

I was proud to bring this aspect of teaching into my school. I felt that now I was truly connecting to the tradition of Taekwondo. At Sigward's, I did not feel this connection because I only taught a simple, generic form of martial art at the request of Mr. Sigward, who wanted the class to have a broad appeal for his members. I was very grateful to him for giving me my start as an instructor, but only in my own school did I begin to feel my life as a master instructor blossom. Taekwondo was truly becoming my path of physical, mental, and spiritual development, and I felt very proud to be bringing this martial art, an art of life, to the United States.

Its newness in this country also brought with it some unique experiences. Numerous times, a visitor would enter the school and ask to observe a class. This was natural and to be expected. Often, prospective students wanted to get a feeling for this particular style of martial art to see if they would like to study. They would observe for half an hour or so, and then I would meet and talk with them for a while; many students came to study with me this way. However, sometimes, people surprised me. I would approach them as usual, but there the familiarity ended.

I remember one such incident vividly.

"Are you Master Chun?" asked a young man. He stood before me with a sense of distance and coldness. Dressed in sweat pants, he was a muscular man, obviously in good shape.

"Yes, I am. Can I help you? Maybe you are here to learn about our school; you can observe a class, if you wish," I said.

"I don't know much about the martial arts," he said. "I am trained as a boxer. How does this martial art compare with boxing?"

"What do you mean, compare?" I said. "There is a great difference." He stood before me with mistrust. "How can I help you?"

"I would like to challenge you—your way of fighting against mine. Now."

This came as a big surprise and, of course, the last thing I wanted to do was fight. I did not want to seem afraid and back down in front of my students who had witnessed the challenge, yet fighting must always be the last resort.

"Why don't you simply observe for a while," I said. "I think that might be better. I'm sure you will learn a lot and if you have any questions or feel that you want more, we can show you a simple demonstration and let you join us for a trial session."

I began to tell him about the structure of the practice session when he interrupted me in the middle of a sentence.

"I did not come here to talk," he said.

I saw that I was not getting anywhere with this line of questioning.

"All right," I said.

I cleared the gym floor to prepare for sparring, hoping that it would never get that far. As soon as we stepped out to the center of the floor, I whirled to face him. His arms rose in boxing position.

I yelled, "ya," in a fearless voice, and went right into a jump kick at lightning speed, returning to fighting position in a split second to do a back kick inches from his face. All this was done before he could even release a punch. The speed overwhelmed and confused him and the confrontation ended without incident. This is how most of these confrontations ended, with these unexpected guests leaving bewildered. Some, however, agreed to stay on to watch the class perform. A number of these confrontations actually led to new students.

One confrontation, which led to many new students, is one that I care not to remember. It actually did not occur in the school. During this time, I attended English classes at Baruch College one night a week. After class one beautiful spring evening, a friend and I decided to take a walk to Greenwich Village. We went into a bar for something to eat and drink. Seated at a table, we were minding our own business when a group of six guys, who looked in their twenties, approached us. One stepped forward.

"Hey, you guys have any change?" he said. "I want to buy a beer but I'm a bit short. Do you mind?"

We thought this was strange, but didn't think too much of it. I went into my pockets and gave the guy three dollars. The group walked out of the bar, but ten minutes later they returned and approached us again.

"Say, we could use some more money. What do you say?"

"But I already gave you some money. I cannot give you more."

"Oh, you're not going to give us any money this time," he said, leaning his head back toward the group.

"We cannot afford to give you money again. We are college students and don't make much ourselves," I said.

"I think you should give us some money," he said, nodding his head arrogantly. All this was taking place quite inconspicuously at our table in the noisy bar. I began to sense trouble.

I leaned over to my friend at the table. "Go over to the corner if something happens," I whispered. Then I stood up and walked over to the bar, leaning against the rail. The group followed me.

"I do not have any more money to give you," I said.

"Oh yeah," said someone who stepped out from the group and reached towards my wrist to grab my watch. Instinctively, I blocked him from getting close. My reaction was spontaneous and natural, but they saw this response only as an invitation to fight. Two closed in on me, and one grabbed me by my belt to lift me up. I quickly pushed him off with a quick hit to the chest. At this point, I decided that I must act first. The situation was getting out of hand quickly, and there were six of them against me. The longer I waited, the more danger I was in. So without warning, using foot and hand techniques, I hit them rapidly and effectively, one in the neck, another directly on the temple, and another on pressure points in the chest. In less than a minute, two of them were down and unconsciousness, while the other four ran off in fear.

In a matter of minutes the police and an ambulance arrived. The two of them were taken to the hospital, while the police questioned me.

"Who are you ? What happened? How did you do this?" they asked.

I told them it was self-defense and that I used martial arts. I was afraid to speak too much because I was the foreigner and I thought that I might be deported. Then I heard.

"He is telling the truth. That group started it and he was just defending himself. That group has caused trouble in here before." It was the bartender coming to my defense; he had seen the whole incident as it occurred at the bar. I was asked to give details and then let go without further involvement, yet the story was not over.

By coincidence, it happened that as the police and ambulance arrived, a reporter from the New York Post passed by the bar. He inquired about the commotion and was given some information. It obviously stirred his interest because the following day a short article came out in the newspaper about a young Korean martial artist, with my name and school mentioned, who defended himself in a Greenwich Village bar against six men who had assaulted him. The article mentioned that the two men, who were taken to the hospital, were released shortly and were not harmed. I was happy to read that. Yet, I had mixed feelings about the whole incident. This was the first time that I had used my martial arts training for real, and afterwards I noticed that it didn't make me feel good. I appreciated its value for self-defense, but I had always been taught that actual fighting must be the last resort. The incident happened, and nothing could be done about it now. I had responded like a true martial artist, and was even somewhat overwhelmed by the power of my actions. The incident stayed with me, and after a while I felt that I needed some closure.

Two weeks later, I stopped by the bar again. By chance, three of the guys who assaulted me were in the bar having a drink. I approached them cautiously, ready to defend myself again if the situation called for it. They turned to me.

"I just wanted to say that I am sorry I hit you at that time. I had no choice," I said.

They just stood there listening.

"I would like to buy you some drinks, if you want," I said.

They nodded. I ordered drinks for them and left right after I paid the bartender. I felt good about what I did and didn't think much about the incident after that.

For several months, the phone in my office would ring with someone on the other end of the line who had read the news story in the paper and now wanted to study martial arts. If you asked me, I would not have wanted it this way, but I did gain at least 15 new students due to that evening in Greenwich Village and the unexpected publicity that it generated.

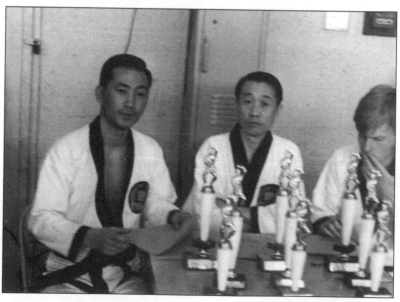

At the promotion test, Silver Spring, MD., 1965. Richard Chun (left) and Grandmaster Ki Whang Kim (right).

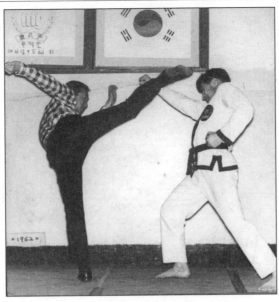

Richard Chun with his top senior student Frank Fuentes at Sigward Sports Academy,
New York City, 1962.

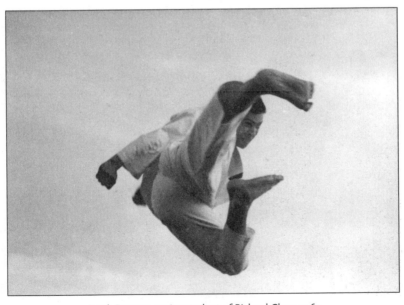

Frank Fuentes, senior student of Richard Chun, 1963.

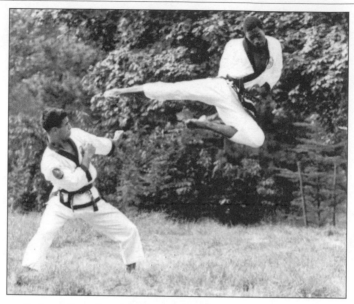

Senior students Joseph Hayes (right) and Frank Fuentes (left), 1964.

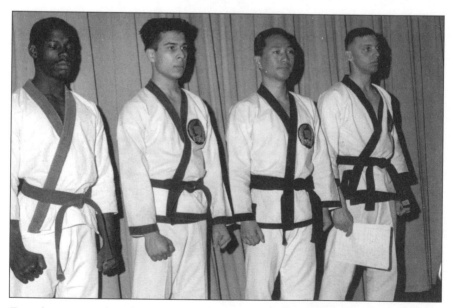

Team demonstration by Richard Dhun Taekwondo Center, New York City, at Fort Dix, New Jersey, 1965. From left to right; Phillip Wargo, Richard Chun, Frank Fuentes, Joseph Hayes.

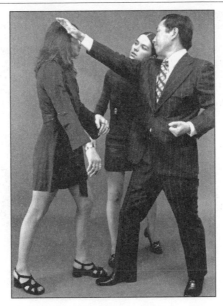

Richard Chun in women's self-defense class.

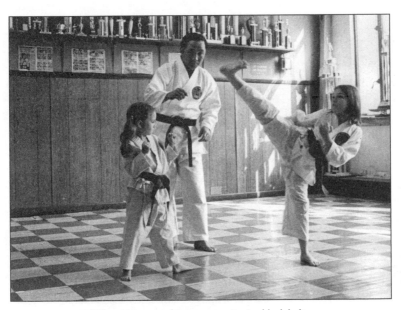

Richard Chun teaching pee wee junior black belts.

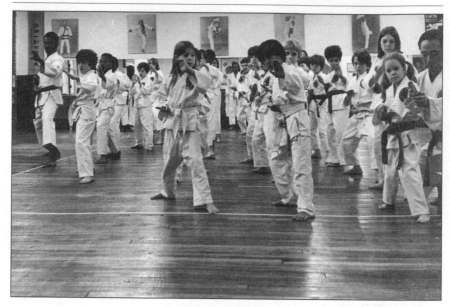

Richard Chun in children's class.

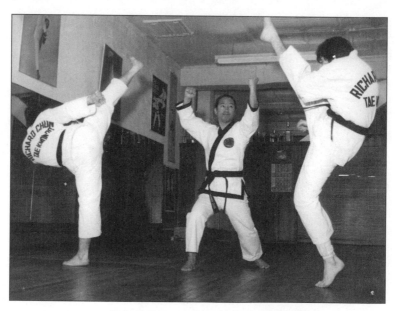

Richard Chun sparring with instructors.

CHAPTER 7

A Decade of Change

One afternoon the phone rang in my office. It was Dr. Kim.

"Annyunghaseyo, Master Chun. Can you have lunch with me tomorrow?"

He sounded excited, almost out of breath. This was uncharacteristic for Dr. Kim. He was usually soft-spoken, always graceful and elegant, always the diplomat.

"Yes, of course Dr. Kim. But what is it? Why are you so excited?" I said.

"I want you to meet someone," he said. "You will see tomorrow. Meet me at 12:30 at Sam Bok.

I hung up the phone. Sam Bok. It was one of the finest Korean restaurants in Manhattan. I wondered what Dr. Kim was up to. Maybe he had found a beautiful Korean woman for me to marry, someone that he thought would be a good match. More than once he had hinted to me that maybe it was time that I found someone and settle down.

"I am not ready yet, Dr. Kim. My life is still developing, too hectic. I don't have the time," I would say. I was serious with my words.

I believe that experiences and events come into a person's life only when you are truly ready for them. It is a natural progression that one cannot force, but only flow along with; there is no other choice, in my opinion. Training in the martial arts taught me this lesson. You may want to develop as a martial artist faster, learn a particular form quicker, perfect a specific punch or kick in a mere few days. However, you realize that your mastery as a martial artist is, in reality, beyond your control. All you can do is train to the best of your ability every day and allow your progress to develop at its own natural pace. You must not be attached to the outcome, but only give yourself—one hundred percent—to the process.

Dr. Kim and I were like brothers. I listened to his advice, but with regards to marriage, I didn't agree with him. Working during the day and running a school at night and on weekends kept me very busy. Marriage and starting a family did not seem right at this time. Yet, I appreciated his advice because I knew he was always thinking of me. Dr. Kim was the most unselfish man I knew. And who knows, maybe Dr. Kim really had found the perfect woman for me. For whatever reason, I looked forward to our lunch.

I immediately arranged to take an extended lunch from my job at IBM "for personal reasons." It would be no problem because I was a reliable and diligent worker, and didn't ask for extra time too often. My boss was understanding and said to take as much time as I needed.

The following day I arrived at Sam Bok promptly at 12:30. As I entered, I was politely greeted by a smiling hostess with short hair. She led me to a table where Dr. Kim was already seated. When he saw me, he stood up and greeted me.

"Master Chun," he said.

I bowed to him. "Who is she?" I asked.

"She?" said Dr. Kim with a puzzled look upon his face. Suddenly, the door to the restaurant opened. Dr. Kim let out a breath and grabbed me by the arm, leading me in the direction of the person who had just entered. He was an American man dressed in a double-breasted gray suit. We approached him.

"Master Chun," Dr. Kim said, "I would like you to meet General James Van Fleet."

My eyes popped open. The General bowed gracefully, familiar with the traditional Korean greeting. General Van Fleet was well known to all Koreans. During the Korean War, he was second in command of the U.S. forces under General Macarthur. In the eyes of the Korean people, he was one of the key men directly responsible for helping keep South Korea a free nation. However, as much as he distinguished himself during the war, it was his work after the war assisting in the rebuilding process that truly distinguished him. He was a popular figure at the time and a true hero to all the Korean people.

"General Van Fleet," I said. "I am honored."

"It is my pleasure," he said in a clear, self-assured tone. "Dr. Kim has spoken highly of you."

The hostess escorted us to our table.

"General Van Fleet and I met when I was in military service during the war," said Dr. Kim. "We actually worked together for a while. Now, he is retired and working as a consultant for business."

We sat and Dr. Kim immediately ordered for us. The exchange of pleasantries continued for a while. During this time, I observed the General closely. He was an imposing figure, combining many interesting qualities. He was a large man over six feet tall and powerfully built. His hair was closely cropped adding to his military character and creating an air of invincibility. At the same time, he was warm and gentle. He smiled constantly, and by his words, you knew that he had a great love for Korea.

"I remember entering a boy's school on the day the war ended to announce our final victory. About a hundred boys surrounded me and cheered like seasoned soldiers. It brought tears to my eyes," said the General.

As he was telling stories, he ate his lunch with great gusto.

"Korea has always been good to me, Master Chun, " he said. "I'm always thinking of ways I can give something in return."

"You have given a great deal already, Sir," I said. " You are a hero to all Koreans."

"General Van Fleet and I were talking about this the other day at the UN," Dr. Kim said. "How to bring more awareness of the Korean culture to the American people."

"That's when your name came up." said General Van Fleet, looking at me.

I cocked my head in surprise. "Me?"

"Yes, we agreed that through the martial arts we are promoting Korean culture," said Dr. Kim.

"Yes, of course," I said.

"That's when we had an idea to further promote Korean culture," Dr. Kim said.

"How?" I asked.

"Dr. Kim actually had the idea," said General Van Fleet, "that we could hold a tournament here in New York for martial artists like nothing that has ever been done before."

My eyes lit up as Dr. Kim and the General explained their idea. They knew that I would respond enthusiastically. We were so engaged in our conversation that I almost forgot we were eating, and by the time dessert and coffee came around, we had already given birth to the idea of the First Universal Open Championship.

In the U.S. at that time, each style of martial art—Korean, Chinese, Japanese—were all separate from each other. Tournaments were held on a small scale between schools of each style, but nothing had been organized to integrate all the martial arts. The First Universal Open Championship would be different because it would be the first to include all styles for all levels as well as matches for women and seniors (martial artists over 35 years of age). Dr. Kim, we decided, would be President of the championship and General Van Fleet an advisor. I was designated as the chief organizer, promoter, and master of ceremonies. As our lunch concluded, we were so excited about the prospect of the tournament that we even congratulated ourselves as we departed company at the restaurant and headed back to our jobs. I walked away from lunch that day as the organizer of what would be one of the largest martial art events in the U.S. at the time.

You can imagine what my life was like during the next 12 months. I worked during the day at IBM, ran my martial art school at night, and now I had to find time to search for and book tournament space, prepare promotional materials, carry out advertising and promotions, and oversee all aspects of the championship. It was both exhausting and exhilarating. I found that I had much energy and everything progressed quite smoothly. Dr. Kim and General Van Fleet, although busy with their government and business responsibilities, gave me constant support and motivation.

In only three months after our lunch, after scouting out numerous possible venues, I placed a deposit on the Manhattan Center located midtown for the championship headquarters. I booked three large rooms: a reception hall to greet and register the participants and guests, a large basement room where we would hold the trials, and a 2000 seat auditorium for the final matches.

Good fortune came at every turn. Thanks to the help of a few students who worked at a printing shop, I was able to produce flyers and posters at a reasonable rate. Armed with these materials, I turned into a non-stop promoter, hiring students to poster throughout the city and at local colleges, attending all martial arts tournaments to speak with masters and putting a plug for the championship. I traveled as far as Washington, DC, where every year a master I knew held an all-city tournament. There, I was able to promote the championship to a large group. In addition, I sent announcements to many martial arts schools in neighboring states and advertised in the local editions of martial arts magazines. I certainly felt that I had all bases covered and soon moved on to the next phase of registering participants. Calls and letters came in from all over the east coast, and it soon became evident that our championship was going to be well attended.

During this time, I was in constant contact with Dr. Kim and General Van Fleet, apprising them of the progress. They were very happy to hear the reports and were working hard themselves to promote the championship. General Van Fleet spoke about it wherever his business took him, and he had arranged for a few celebrities to come as special guests. Dr. Kim often contacted government officials as part of his work for the UN, and he was promoting the championship here and in Korea.

Upon returning from one of his trips to Korea, he showed up at the school in the middle of a practice session with a large box in his hand. He occasionally brought back gifts from Korea for his friends and co-workers, so I didn't think much of it. That evening, however, he gestured for me to come over right away to see him. I interrupted the lesson at an appropriate time and approached him.

"Dr. Kim, you are back from your trip. It is good to see you. What do you have there?" I said.

"Come here," said Dr. Kim, "I want to show you something."

He led me into my office and shut the door behind him. Placing the box on the table, he cut the tape with a pair of scissors and pulled out an object wrapped in newspaper.

"It's a gift from the Blue House," he said. The Blue House was the name for the Presidential offices in Seoul. He unwrapped it like a child on Christmas morning and held it out for me to see: a beautiful trophy of a martial arts figure in kicking position on a solid wood base. A bronze plaque on the base read:

1967
First Universal Open Championship

To: Richard Chun
In Appreciation and For
Your Successful Tournament
New York City

From: the Blue House
Seoul, Korea

"It's beautiful," I cried out.

"That's not all," Dr. Kim said. "Many dignitaries and officials from the government offices are donating trophies for the championship."

We were both so happy that we started to laugh.

"Many friends in Korea are supporting our tournament," he said.

I took the trophy out of Dr. Kim's hands. "I must show this to the students," I said.

"Yes," said Dr. Kim, "maybe it will inspire one of your students to win."

The year of organization and preparations quickly drew to a close. With only one week remaining, everything was in place. Over 450 participants had registered from every style of martial art, and we were expecting close to 2000 spectators. Many students from my school and other schools from the area volunteered their time to prepare the hall and assist during the championship. We officially opened the doors the day before the matches to greet the participants and hold a brief meeting to explain the rules and logistics of the championship day. We all gathered in the auditorium. Dr. Kim, General Van Fleet and I sat on stage along with the referees and judges who were masters and owners of martial arts schools in the area.

I spoke first, greeting the participants and introducing the judges. Then, Dr. Kim stood and introduced General Van Fleet. The General spoke briefly, praising the participants and wishing them good luck in their matches. Then, I explained the rules and regulations of the tournament.

"Different martial art styles will compete together," I said. "The matches will be scored on a non-contact point system. You will be required to stop your move just before a hit. The referee will stop the match if he perceives a legal hit. Points will be awarded by a majority rule by the judges. In the event of a split decision, the referee will break the tie. Any intentional contact will result in disqualification. The matches will be two minutes in length. Any questions?"

There were none. So, I concluded.

"It will be a long day tomorrow. Please go home or back to your hotels and get good rest today, and good luck in your competition tomorrow."

That evening I slept lightly in anticipation of the next day. All my work during the past year had been focused on a single day—tomorrow—the championship day. Everything was now out of my hands. The day would go fine, I assured myself. Everything was in place, and by tomorrow night, I would surely be feeling the fruits of my work. Eventually, I drifted off to sleep only to be awoken early in the morning to the phone ringing. It's starting already, I thought. I answered, reluctantly, and to my surprise it was the Korean ambassador calling to wish me success for the day and to thank me for organizing such an event.

"Thank you, Mr. Ambassador," I said in a sleepy voice, "but the day has hardly begun."

I arrived at the Manhattan Center at 6:00 AM. The trials were scheduled to begin at 9:00. Already the place was full of excitement and activity. I greeted many people whom I had met during the past year. The morning's events would take place in the lower hall. It was covered wall to wall with mats. Ten matches would take place simultaneously. We calculated that by mid-afternoon the trials would be completed. After a break, we would begin the final matches on the stage upstairs in the auditorium. When the first set of trial matches began, I truly felt as if I were letting go. The championships had begun. From this point on it was out of my hands and into the hands of the martial artists who were performing.

The trials went smoothly and perfectly. By 5:00 PM, the 450 participants were narrowed down to 36. Soon, the finals would begin.

Nine of my students had made it this far, six in non-black belt matches and three in the black belt division. One of my students, Joe Hayes, was in one of the most anticipated matches of the day: the lightweight, black belt match. Joe was my best student. He had an incredible blend of speed and strength, intimidating and overwhelming his opponents with his presence and power. He was the favorite to win.

When the finals began, we all moved to the upper stage. Each match took place on the stage, one at a time, with the spectators seated in the auditorium, looking upward at them like at the theater. The organizers, special guests and celebrities, including General Van Fleet, Dr. Kim, senior masters, judges, and referees were all seated on the stage. They were introduced and General Van Fleet welcomed the contestants and spectators. Then, I welcomed everyone and thanked the General, Dr. Kim, the judges, and referees for their work. After explaining the rules of the tournament, I gave a 15-minute demonstration on self-defense against attacks with weapons with 5 of my black belt students. The audience liked it very much and gave us a standing ovation. Then the final matches began.

Right from the start the performances were exceptional. The fourth match, middleweight green belt, pitted a young Filipino fighting in his country's style against one of my students using Taekwondo. The match started out even, each fighter trading a blow and a point. Then, the Filipino's speed got the best of my student and he lost two quick points. The match ended 5 to 2, my student losing. My second student, a red belt, also lost his match to a very powerful martial artist practiced in Taekwondo. Despite their losses, I was proud of their accomplishments. As the finals continued, the tension and excitement in the auditorium increased because the fighters were more adept and advanced. Finally, it was time for the Grand Champion Title Match of the day. To get to this match, the three weight divisions in black belt—light, middle, and heavy—fight each other in a round robin competition. In the final match, Joe Hayes, lightweight champion fighting Taekwondo faced a very strong heavyweight fighter using a Japanese form of Karate.

It was a very proud moment for me personally for many reasons. The tournament was like my baby and now my prime student was about to perform. I felt that Joe, in the final match of the tournament, was like a reflection of me and my work as a master and organizer in the martial arts. I felt nervous and proud, like a father. This feeling was new to me, yet I would soon come to know it well through all my experiences as a martial artist. There was nothing I took more seriously than my ability and responsibility to pass on the tradition. Each student became a reflection of myself. Joe was my first student who had risen to such heights.

The match began. For the first minute, each competitor traded a few moves but no points were awarded. It seemed that they were just sizing each other up. Then, Joe's opponent scored quickly on an upper body punch. Being scored against first could be devastating for a young student. It could cause a loss of concentration and ultimately lead to defeat in the match. However, being hit first only seemed to motivate Joe. He executed a series of punches, scoring no points; however, I knew that this was a decoy because he was setting up for his turning jump kick. I was familiar with his routine. He began to execute his kick with lightning speed when his opponent, not realizing the kick was even in progress, stepped in to execute a punch and walked right into the kick. He was knocked to the floor with great force but was not hurt. However, since contact was made, there was question whether or not Joe would be disqualified. I sat on the edge of my seat and held my breath. The referee stopped the match to consult with the judges. During those moments, a hush filled the auditorium. After a couple of minutes the judges made an announcement, ruling that contact had been unavoidable. The opponent had entered into Joe's space while he was in mid-air and therefore could not stop his move. I let out a deep breath. It was a good call and Joe had been saved; the incident also seemed to give Joe a temporary edge over his opponent. In the next minute, he scored two points with a series of kicks followed with punches. His opponent recovered with a quick hit. Then, Joe scored again on a powerful turning hook kick that took his opponent off guard. Joe was on his way to victory. The score ended 5 to 2. Joe Hayes had become grand champion.

When the judges called the match, I cheered like a young boy at a baseball game. Simultaneously, I felt a sort of let down knowing that the championship, which had consumed one year of my life and brought many good experiences, was over. That feeling passed, however, and I went to Joe and gave him my heartfelt congratulations and a big hug.

That evening, after an inspiring awards ceremony, during which Dr. Kim called the championship "the largest and most successful martial arts gathering in the U.S.," I left the hall with Joe. Everyone congratulated him, patting him on the back as we walked out. He carried his trophy with the help of a friend. It was literally 8 feet tall, a large silver cup on top of a wooden pedestal surrounded with columns. The Korean government donated the trophy. It was a great day for him, myself, and for the martial arts in general.

Joe's star as a martial artist continued to shine bright over the next few years. He won many tournaments and trophies, and progressed inwardly as a martial artist. Both as a student in the martial arts and as a person, Joe had come a long way. He had started with me when he was only 16 years old, a city kid from gang-infested streets, a bit on the rough side. His father had died years before and Joe took on the responsibility of caring for his grandfather while going to school. When Joe came to me, he was a young kid with lots of emotion and potential, but his energy needed channeling and discipline. Joe immediately took to his martial arts training and appreciated my stern and disciplined manner. I took him under my wing and soon became like a second father to him. As he developed as a martial artist, I also felt a fatherly pride in his accomplishments. However, an unfortunate incident took place some years after the championship that changed his life forever.

One evening, Joe was driving on a highway when his car got a flat tire. He pulled over to change the flat and a police car pulled up behind him. A friendly officer approached and offered to help, which Joe accepted. At one point, Joe went to look for a flashlight in the glove compartment as the policeman started taking off the wheel. In that instant, a passing car lost control and swerved too close, hitting the policeman and killing him instantly. Joe saw the policeman die right in front of him. Joe was severely shaken and depressed by the incident and never returned to his practice in the martial arts. In the aftermath of the tragedy, he began to question the events in his life and began to seek a deeper meaning in these experiences. He became a more religious man during this time and eventually became a missionary.

Over the years, Joe has put this traumatic incident in perspective. He now leads a happy, healthy life with his family in Rockwall, Texas, as a coach at a local high school and a missionary in a church. We have remained friends and talk over the phone occasionally even to this day. Recently, he mentioned to me that during his years of training under me he learned the value of humility and respect for tradition, teachers, elders, and God.

"I still carry that with me," he said.

In my eyes, Joe will always be a champion and certainly one of my best students ever.

As far as The First Universal Open Championships were concerned, it was a great success and for months afterwards I received numerous letters and phone calls from participants, spectators, and judges thanking me for organizing the event. Everyone requested that I make it an annual one. Considering the time it took me to feel fully recovered and rested, I was uncertain about an annual event. However, a few months after the championship, Dr. Kim, General Van Fleet, and I met again for lunch. Over lunch, we toasted our success with champagne. When I told them about the responses we received, the discussion of another championship began. It did not take long to decide that we would do it again next year. As it turned out, that next year turned into an annual event for the next ten years.

I was able to cut the organizational process down from one year to three months. Each year we grew, so we consciously kept a limit on the numbers to insure manageability and quality. We intended to keep the championship a one-day event.

The more subtle effects of the championships were not evident until a few years later. They brought enormous changes to my life. The practice of the martial arts in the U.S. was enjoying a great rise in popularity. Many students of Taekwondo, whom I had trained and met throughout the years, had progressed to black belt. A number of them had moved to different parts of the country, as their lives led them, and opened their own martial art schools. I began to receive invitations from these students to visit their schools to inspire their students, many of whom had never met a Korean master, and consult with them on how to organize a tournament for their city or state. I was happy to oblige. So, a few times a year I began traveling around the country to cities like Miami, Atlanta, Dallas, San Diego, Chicago, Los Angeles, and San Juan to meet with my former students and their students.

These trips were very enjoyable. Not only was I promoting Taekwondo more than ever, but I was seeing the United States for the first time. It was during these ten years that martial arts in the U.S. exploded across the country and has remained popular ever since.

On one trip I went to visit a former student in Las Vegas. After a meeting and demonstration with his students, we decided to have dinner at a restaurant in a nearby casino. While seated at our table, I spotted another former student of mine, Gregory Hines, who was pursuing a career as a performer. When he was first starting out in show business, a small act with his father and brother, he studied with me and progressed quickly to black belt. He was an excellent martial artist—disciplined, athletic and limber—due to his dance training. We greeted each other warmly and I invited him to join us at our table.

"Grandmaster Chun, what are you doing in Las Vegas?" he asked.

I told him about the championships over the past few years and my travels visiting former students across the country. He was happy and excited about it.

"How are you?" I asked. "How is your career?"

He looked happy, but tired.

"Oh, it's all right," he said, "but very difficult. I'm working very hard to establish myself. It's non-stop. Sometimes I don't know if I'm going to make it. And I see others around me who have achieved success so quickly and easily."

Always the teacher, I told him "be patient and believe in yourself. The time will come for your success."

He nodded in agreement and understanding. These were words he heard before as my student in the martial arts. I always impressed upon my students that they could accomplish any goal, but only through hard work and believing in oneself. There would be times of struggle and hardship. During these times, particularly, it was crucial to not give up, but reaffirm your beliefs and desires, and stick to your goal. I reminded Gregory of these points.

"You must have strong conviction and persistence. Stick to your goal. Remember, this is what I taught you during your training as a martial artist. And, never compare yourself to others who have had early success. There is a time and place for everyone. Yours will come."

"You are right, Grandmaster Chun," he said. "I know this. In fact, I believe my practice in the martial arts has given me the courage and strength to continue even when I don't completely trust in myself. "

"I'm sure you will succeed," I said.

While I was in Las Vegas, Gregory and I saw each other one more times. During our meeting, he casually introduced me to an executive at NBC who, to my surprise, some months later called me to ask if I would like to appear on the Johnny Carson Show. Martial arts, particularly Taekwondo, were enjoying increased popularity and the producers agreed that it would be entertaining to have a Grandmaster in the martial arts as a guest on the show. They were hoping for a specific date the following month.

I was excited about the prospect, but unfortunately I had a prior commitment in Korea to conduct business with the World Taekwondo Federation and the Moo Duk Kwan Association. However, I did suggest that someone could represent me and the art of Taekwondo. I immediately called Gregory, told him the news, and he happily agreed to appear on the show on my behalf.

One month later, Gregory was on National TV sitting next to Johnny Carson and his co-host, Ed McMahon. Johnny was his customary self, friendly and funny, but he also treated people with sincerity and respect. I liked that combination. Gregory was at ease.

He sat and answered questions about Taekwondo, his training, and he told stories about me as his Korean Grandmaster. Johnny made a few jokes about his bare feet and then asked him to demonstrate a few moves. Gregory went over to an open area on the set and performed some advanced kicking and breaking techniques. Every time he yelled out "ya," the audience burst out in cheers. Then, Johnny came over dressed in a dobok over his suit, looking comical, and wanted Gregory to instruct him in some breaking techniques. First, Gregory illustrated some punching and kicking moves and Johnny followed. Then, Johnny broke some boards with punches and kicks. Whenever he broke a board, the audience went wild. Finally, Gregory presented Johnny with an honorary black belt and black belt certificate on my behalf.

They went back to their seats and the conversation continued.

"Does your teacher, Master Chun, ever want to leave teaching and go into the movies? Has he ever been approached by directors?" Johnny asked Gregory.

"Oh yes," he said, which was true. "Movie producers and directors from

Hong Kong have approached Grandmaster Chun. Hong Kong is where many martial art pictures are made."

"And," asked Johnny.

"He refused," Gregory said and the audience let out a disappointed moan.

"Why?" questioned Johnny. "He could make a million dollars, retire early, and spend the rest of his life resting his sore muscles." He made a gesture indicating that during his demonstration he had pulled a muscle. The audience laughed.

"In order to make a movie in Hong Kong, he would have to leave New York and his school for six months at a time. Grandmaster Chun loves his school and his teaching. So unfortunately for us moviegoers, we miss seeing a great martial artist in action, but fortunately for us students, we have a great master available."

The audience clapped upon hearing Gregory tell that I chose to stick to what I felt in my heart.

"Does Grandmaster Chun know Bruce Lee and Chuck Norris?" asked Johnny.

"They both have met him at several tournaments to exchange ideas and techniques. I know that they are excellent martial artists and are becoming good actors, too."

The segment finally ended and all agreed that it was a great success. I was forever indebted to Gregory for appearing on the show. And, regarding Gregory's career, success did come to him. Years later, Gregory was back in New York as the star of a Broadway show. His career as a performer has never waned since.

One evening, I went to the theater with some friends to see Gregory, planning to go backstage to say hello before the show. I didn't know that the correct protocol was to see the star after the show, and not before. Therefore, the security guard would not allow us to see Gregory. I left my card with the security guard and asked him to please give it to Gregory. We enjoyed the show and afterwards went home, not knowing that Gregory had cleared my way for us to come backstage for an after-show visit. The following morning Gregory called me to ask why I hadn't come to see him; he had waited for a while with the entire cast to meet me. I was deeply touched by his gesture. Such is the strong bond that is created between student and teacher.

Over the next ten years, my influence grew enormously in the world of the martial arts, and the world of the martial arts grew enormously in size. I felt as if I had been put in the right place at the right time. Other forces of change were also working upon me. Having an MBA in marketing, I was enjoying my job with IBM in the Department of Marketing Research and Planning; I was learning quite a lot about advanced market research techniques. Often, I gave seminars to Korean businessmen who were interested in expanding their businesses, both domestic and international.

These businessmen as well as others based in Korea were interested in opening their markets in the U.S., and a need arose for someone to help study Korean market potential in the U.S. Due to my connection with Korean businessmen, I was the obvious person. Therefore, I decided to leave my job at IBM and devote myself full-time to Korean market research and promoting the martial arts.

I started a company called the Korean Marketing and Research Corporation, working for Korean companies. The timing was perfect; it was another example of an opportunity coming along just at the right time. All was ripe for success, and the business grew quickly. I even began to get accounts from the Korean government. It was now about seven years after the first championship. My school was still going strong and I was still chief organizer of the annual championships, yet with my new company and added responsibilities, I was unsure how long I could continue being part of the championship tournament.

At this time, in the mid 1970's, the Korean economy was struggling, still shaking off the remnants of the war. However, it was given a huge boost by winning large construction bids in the oil-rich Middle Eastern countries. Hundreds of thousands of Koreans were employed in these countries and millions of dollars exchanged. I began working for one of the largest construction companies in Korea, providing them with the best and most reliable manufacturers of aluminum windows, curtain walls, and other related construction products.

My school, by this time, was well established. I had trained a number of strong black belts to assist me in my teaching responsibilities. That freed up time for this new business venture. My daily routine was to spend the early part of the day at the school, taking care of daily business and seeing that everything was functioning. Then, I did my market research work out of a friend's office on Park Avenue. In a few years, my responsibilities with the school and business became too full for me to organize the annual championships. After ten successful years as organizer, I gave up that responsibility. Unfortunately, no one else stepped into the position and the Universal Open Championships finally came to an end.

During these years, I also often traveled to Korea and the Middle East, sometimes staying for a month at a time, to follow-up on business transactions. I discovered that I enjoyed the traveling and business very much. It was a completely different world from the martial arts, but many of the tactics that I used as a martial artist were also appropriate in the business field. I was able to apply my Taekwondo training to my marketing business. Most obvious to me was the patience and determination needed to see a business deal through to the end. I had learned these qualities quite strongly through my training in the martial arts. The patience and determination required to master a complex black belt form is the same as that required to make numerous phone calls and go through numerous negotiations all so a large supply of products can be shipped from the U.S. to Kuwait via a Korean merchant.

Less obvious, but maybe more powerful, was the growing mastery of self that I began to feel doing business. The deepest result of being a martial artist is the sense of mastery of self that gradually develops in one's life. I found that I had a clear vision of my purpose in this new business and a sharp insight into the nuances of its inner workings. I began to feel invincible in my business deals. I also felt that I was providing a good and just service. The sheer energy and focus that the business demanded was readily available in order to keep pace with the daily events, to flow with unexpected twists and turns of business, or to deal with unforeseen mishaps or problems. Although the work was tiring at times, I felt that things were under control.

After several years of running this successful business, the construction boom in the Middle Eastern countries began to wane due to the world oil crisis and the lowering of oil prices. These countries could no longer afford to carry out their elaborate construction plans. As a result, I decided to slow down the marketing business and go back to school to further my studies. At that time, I was teaching several courses at Hunter College, City University of New York, as Associate Professor in the Department of Health and Physical Education. I wanted to get a degree in Education.

After receiving my Ph.D., I began teaching courses at Hunter and other colleges and universities in the New York area on sports psychology, physical & health education and the martial arts. I also spent more time teaching black belts from all over the world. My name in the martial art field, by now, was becoming well known and often I traveled, by invitation or business, to different countries. Wherever I went I was invited to give classes to advanced students at local martial art schools.

I began to feel, finally, that life was settling down for me, even though I was still very active. I think focusing upon education and teaching created the desire to express myself and my experiences more. During this time, I began work on my first book on Taekwondo. It would be a basic how-to-book covering the fundamental philosophy and providing descriptions of forms and techniques required to achieve a certain level of mastery.

After I finished writing, two books emerged: "*Tae Kwon Do: Korean Martial Art*" and "*Advancing In Tae Kwon Do*," both published by Harper Collins. Other books that eventually followed were "*Tae Kwon Do—Moo Duk Kwan*", Volume I and II, published by Ohara Publications, a martial arts publisher based in California, and a series of Tae Kwon Do home study videotapes. This was an interesting time for me, seeing my knowledge enjoyed by all those who had an interest in the martial arts and Taekwondo.

We must trust in nature's grand plan to bring us the right things in our lives at the right time. This is the heart and soul of a martial artist. My period of writing came right after an intense fifteen years of activity doing my part to help popularize martial arts in this country, organizing the open championships, and then becoming involved in an exciting business venture.

Even now, I continue to write and am presently working on a book for woman's self-defense, tentatively titled "*Fight Back: A Manual Of Self-Defense For Women.*"

As the years passed, I remained involved in some business apart from my school. In the mid 1980's, I became involved in importing leather goods, such as jackets, boots, and gloves from Korea and China for motorcyclists. I continued this business for several years but then decided to devote all my time to training and educating others in the martial arts. This was the home that I have always come back to.

Whatever business endeavors I encountered or created, I have only my training as a martial artist to thank for giving me the strength and confidence to pursue them.

During all these years, Dr. Kim and General Van Fleet were still active in the martial arts. General Van Fleet continued to lend his name to the championships and other events, but his business and health kept him from attending. Dr. Kim, on the other hand, became very well known and influential in the world of Taekwondo. He left his post at the Korean embassy and moved back to Korea to work in the office of the President. Simultaneously, he was chosen to head an organization in Seoul to promote Taekwondo worldwide, known as the World Taekwondo Federation. Again, we found ourselves in constant contact since much of the activity was in the states. His goal for the hundreds of masters and teachers teaching Taekwondo in the U.S. was to unite them in principle and spirit. This was not a simple task, knowing the strong wills and varied natures of the martial artists. He visited a few times a year on official government business but his first priority would always be to meet with the Taekwondo masters.

Usually, I received a call about a month before his arrival.

"Master Chun, I will be in New York one month from today."

I knew what that meant. For the next few days, I called about 50 Taekwondo masters with their own schools to inform them of Dr. Kim's visit. They, in turn, would call other masters, and in a week the news spread that Dr. Kim would be in New York to meet them at a particular location and date. Whoever could attend would travel for a day's discussion with Dr. Kim on the latest news and ideas for promoting Taekwondo.

His main goal, however, was to unite and inspire us with the common vision of adhering to the classical tradition of our art.

I always felt that he was the perfect man for the job. He was well respected among martial artists, a government official and not an owner of a school, he was removed enough from the martial artists to ease their minds. He was clearly not out to satisfy his own needs. Therefore, no one felt threatened by him. Instead, we all felt that he was truly looking out for our best interests. Dr. Kim was always a consummate diplomat.

In recent years, it was due to the work of Dr. Kim that Taekwondo was chosen as a demonstration sport for the 1988 Olympics in Seoul, Korea and the 1992 Olympics in Barcelona, Spain. For a sport to be officially recognized and accepted in the Olympics, it must first appear in the games as a demonstration sport only. The host country, if they wish, may choose a sport to be the demonstration sport for that Olympic year. Of course, when the 1988 Olympics were in Seoul, Taekwondo was the obvious choice. After a number of trials as a demonstration sport, the sport is either accepted or not by the Olympic Committee. Taekwondo performed successfully as a demonstration sport for the past two Olympics. It will now appear as an official sport for the first time in Olympic history in the 2000 Olympics in Sydney, Australia.

While organizing for Taekwondo's introduction into the Olympic games as an official sport for the first time, Dr. Kim also served as Vice President of the International Olympic Committee, as well as President of the General Association of International Sports Federation, which deals with non-Olympic sports. He also finds time to fulfill his responsibilities as I. O. C. Member of Korea, President of the Korean Amateur Sports Association, President of the World Taekwondo Federation, and President of Kukkiwon (World Taekwondo Center).

Dr. Kim has boundless energy and vision, and is truly a modern-day hero in the world of sports. In my mind, it is as a person, a whole human being, where Dr. Kim has truly made his mark. He has always been the perfect embodiment of the enlightened martial artist. Wherever he goes and whatever he does, he inspires people with his graceful presence, self-assurance, dignity, humility, innumerable skills and talents, and long, long list of life-achievements. I consider it a blessing that Dr. Kim has come into my life.

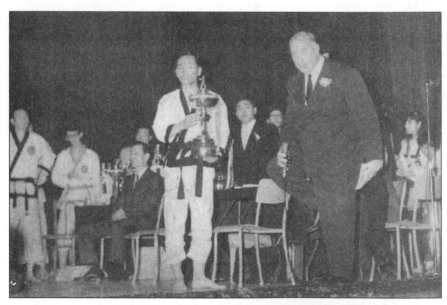

Receiving a silver trophy awarded by the government of Korea, Richard Chun (center). From right, General James Van Fleet; Dr. Un Yong Kim, president of World Taekwondo Federation; Grandmaster Duk Sung Son; Grandmaster Ki Whang Kim at the first Universal Taekwondo Championships, New York City, 1967.

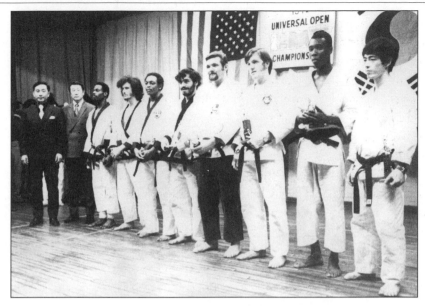

1970 Universal Tournament of Champions. Right to left, Toyotaro Myazaki, Byron Jones, Jeffrey Smith, Bob Engle, Hector Eugui, Jr., Robert Cunningham, Joe Corey, Grand Grand Champion Joseph Hayes, Grandmaster Ki Whang Kim, Richard Chun.

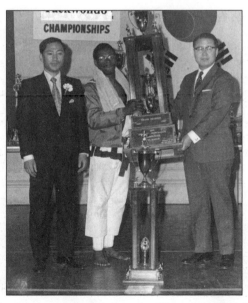

Grand Champion of 1969 Universal Open Taekwondo, Karate, Kung Fu Championships, New York City, 1969. Joseph Hayes, Richard Chun, Ambassador Kyu Sup Chung (right).

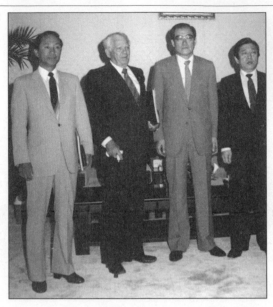

At the award ceremony, from the right, Dr. Un Yong Kim, president of the World Taekwondo Federation & I. O. C. member; Honorable Sung Bae Kim, mayor of Seoul; Honorable German Rieckehoff, chairman of Caribbean Olympic Committee; and Richard Chun, receiving a special award for promoting the art of Taekwondo as a world and Olympic sport, Seoul, Korea, May, 1982.

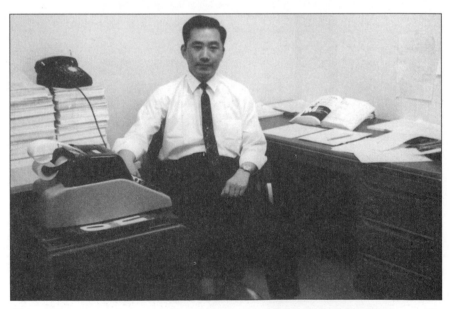

Richard Chun as a marketing research and planning consultant at IBM World Trade Corp., 1966.

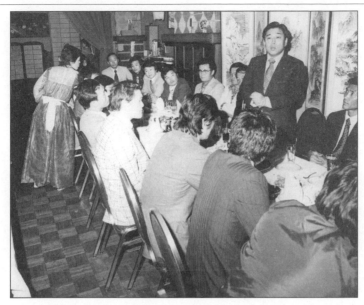

Dr. Un Yong Kim, president of the World Taekwondo Federation, speaking to master instructors, New York City, 1970's.

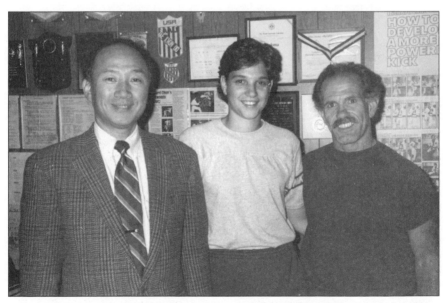

Richard Chun with actor Ralph Macchio and master Pat Johnson at USTA headquarters, after rehearsing for action shooting of the movie *Karate Kid*.

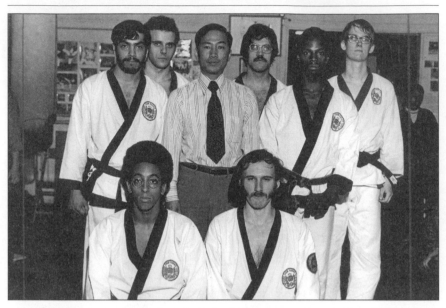

At the promotion test in March, 1969, Richard Chun (center), Gregory Hines (front left).

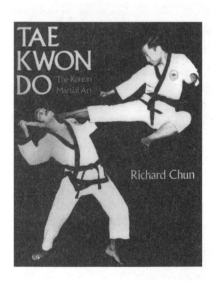

Cover of Richard Chun's first book, *Tae Kwon Do*, 1976. Four more books have been published since.

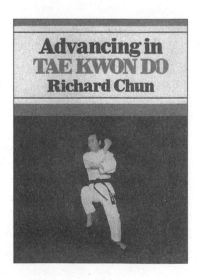

Cover of Richard Chun's second book, 1982.

CHAPTER 8

Birthplace of a Tradition

A letter from Korea arrived in my office in late 1972 announcing the First World Taekwondo Championships to be held the following summer in Seoul. I had been waiting for this announcement to come. On a recent visit by Dr. Kim to New York, he had mentioned to me that he had raised the idea of the championship with the Korean Taekwondo Association about six months ago. The championship would bring together the best Taekwondo martial artists from all around the world. I was happy to see that his idea had come to fruition. The United States would have to be represented, of course. However, there were obstacles to prevent us from sending a team to Korea. Dr. Kim and I had spoken about it previously.

"At the present time, we have no source of funding to form a team. How could we possibly finance such a trip?" I questioned him.

The martial arts, particularly Taekwondo, were gaining in popularity across the U.S. at that time. There were over several hundred schools in Taekwondo, as well as many university and college martial art clubs, yet, it still was not officially recognized as a sport in this country. Therefore, no A.A.U. funding was available for the martial arts as there was for other sports like track and field, basketball, and baseball, sports that had firm roots in American soil. Taekwondo was still considered too foreign. To further complicate the matter, the Taekwondo schools that were in existence were not united or organized in any coherent way. What process could we use to select the best team to represent the U.S.? How could we do it fairly, without overlooking many excellent martial artists? These were the questions that presented themselves to us at that time.

Despite these obstacles, I was determined to see that we be represented in Korea that summer. I decided to let the problem rest for a while after receiving the announcement to see what would develop. Who knows, maybe some unforeseen solutions would present themselves.

A few weeks later, I received a call from Professor Min, a Physical Education Professor at the University of California at Berkeley. He had also received the announcement and had been pondering the same questions as I.

"It is very important that we send a team this spring, Master Chun," said Professor Min. "We have grown so much in this country. It would be a shame if we were not represented."

"Of course, Professor Min," I said.

This began a serious discussion on how to fulfill our desire, no matter what obstacles stood in our way. After a few conversations over the next few days, we decided to contact all the recognized Korean Taekwondo masters in the country, which at that time numbered about twenty-five.

"Hello, this is Master Chun from New York calling. Professor Min and I have been discussing the possibility of forming a team to represent the U.S. at the First World Tae Kwon Championships this spring in Seoul."

With these calls, we opened up two to three busy weeks of animated telephone discussions with masters from around the country. By the end of the month, we had come to a decision. The team members would be black belts hand picked by the masters based on their achievements in tournaments and their reputation in their school. Nominations were sent to a board comprised of seven masters from the largest cities and schools. I was among the seven. The board would have the final say on choosing the team members. In addition, each master would hold a benefit at their school to raise money to sponsor the team.

The next few months brought a whirlwind of activity in our quest to form the teams. Considering the task, it went relatively smoothly. After a few minor disputes over who to choose, we had worked our way down to the final fifteen. There were, of course, disappointments both to the martial artists who were not chosen and to the masters who had wanted their students to be part of the team. Even I had been disappointed. A very strong student of mine in a lower weight class had not been picked. My best student, Joe Hayes, had made the team and in fact was chosen as the team captain. All who were chosen were accomplished black belts from their area and the masters all agreed that we were sending a strong team to Seoul.

The benefits did raise some money, but not enough to sponsor the teams and coaches on a trip to Seoul for ten days. The remainder of the funding actually came out of our pockets, particularly Master Hwang who owned a successful school in Oklahoma. He donated about 25 percent of the expenses for the U.S. teams to be represented.

Our next task was to choose team leaders. Again, a flurry of activity was created with many phone conversations. This time, although hectic, it was quite amusing. The phone rang constantly.

"Master Chun, this is Professor Min. I think Master Hwang would be the best choice for team leader because..."

"Master Chun, this is Master Kim. I think Master Kang would be the best choice for team leader because..."

After a week or two, we finally agreed that Master Hwang would be overall team leader since he was the chief sponsor. He also took on the responsibility of registering the teams for the championship and making all the hotel and travel arrangements. Master Kang, from Sacramento, California, was chosen as team manager. He was the senior among us and his responsibility was as a communication link between the U.S. team and the Korean Taekwondo Association. Professor Min was chosen as assistant manager and Master Ahn, from Dallas, Texas, as co-leader of the team. I was chosen as Head Coach. My responsibility was to train and prepare the team for the competition. I choose two assistant coaches, Master Il Hoi Kim from Harrisburg, Pennsylvania and Master Dae Hyun Kim from Brooklyn, New York to help me.

By early spring, everything was in place. We had formed the teams and selected leaders and coaches. The U.S. would be represented at the First World Taekwondo Championships. Now, it was time to prepare them for competition. This was not an easy task since I would meet the team members as a whole only three days before leaving for Korea. We were all planning to assemble in Los Angeles before departing for Seoul. A month before our departure, to introduce myself to all the team members, I wrote a warm, congratulatory letter to them. There was no need to boost their morale or provide inspiring words. These were serious students of the martial arts, all black belts with years of experience, and they were excited about the prospect of competing in Korea, the birthplace of Taekwondo. For all of the team members, it would be their first trip there.

Throughout the spring, I kept very busy teaching at numerous locations: martial arts at my school, a class on Health and Physical Education at Hunter College of the City University of New York, and seminars on personal development and self-confidence at the Katherine Gibbs School of New York. Before I knew it, the month of May had arrived and I was on my way with a small east coast contingent to Los Angeles for three days of preparation, then on to the championships in Seoul. We would meet the remainder of our delegation in Los Angeles. On the night we arrived, it was hot and sticky, but our spirits were light and soaring. At dinner, the team members, leaders, and coaches met each other for the first time; the conversation centered around nothing but the upcoming championships.

"There will be 22 countries represented in Korea," said Master Hwang.

"I wonder how we will do," said a team member from Pennsylvania.

"The Korean team will be tough," responded another.

"Just being in Korea will be an answer to my prayers," said Joe Hayes.

"We will have much preparation to do beforehand," I interjected.

They all agreed.

"Tomorrow morning we will meet in the second floor conference room for a workout," I said. "I think for now, we should all take a little walk together—there's a beautiful garden just outside—and then get some good rest."

"A fine idea," said Professor Min.

By the end of the evening, we all felt like a family. It was a wonderful experience, and I knew that whatever the championship would bring, the whole experience for us would be a memorable one. For myself, I hadn't been to Korea in a few years and I was very much looking forward to being there. For the team, I knew the experience for them, aside from the actual championship, would be one of great self-discovery. These were the best students from a western country who had risen to become martial artists from an eastern tradition. They were from all walks of life: a teacher, a mechanic, a salesman, a florist, a young executive—all brought together by their love for the sport and art of Taekwondo. Such a diverse group of individuals from all backgrounds and regions of the U.S., all walking down the same path, all tied together with a common bond. There seemed to be a familiarity with each other that transcended the surface, something deeper. I found this to be very interesting, a sort of miracle.

In the Buddhist tradition, which is a very prevalent philosophy in the East, there is a concept known as Karma. Karma is the law of cause and effect in our lives. It is the sum total of all our past actions all which inevitably leads us to where we are today. According to Buddhist tradition, these past actions also include actions from our innumerable past lives. We can't escape our Karma, and inevitably we are drawn back to familiar paths that we have walked down before and to the same people we have known before. Now, I'm not sure of the validity of Karma, but I couldn't help wondering, from the closeness we all had with each other, if we as a group had not been together before in a different time and place.

By 9:00 AM the following morning, the team was assembled in a conference room. It was bare and empty, ready to accommodate a workout for a group of black belts.

When I entered with the assistant coaches and other team leaders, the team members stood at attention, at full alert like military men, and each had wide smiles on their faces, which glowed with anticipation.

"I know that you are as excited as we are," I said, gesturing to myself, the assistant coaches, and the other team leaders that were present. "This will be the start of our journey—the first U.S. Taekwondo team to compete in Korea."

Their smiles seemed to grow even wider.

"We will do our best to prepare you during these three days together before we depart. But, what is most important, I believe, and what I request from all of you, is just to get proper rest during these days. This will contribute towards strong mental training."

I have always believed that proper rest is the basis for successful, dynamic activity. Without a clear, fresh mind, all the training in the world will dissipate before you like a puff of smoke. With proper rest, the mind is sharp and awake, ready to perceive and react, and the coordination between the mind and body naturally more attuned. These ten martial artists had trained hard over the years, each distinguishing themselves and advancing to black belts. I thought that the best preparation for the championship that I could impart to them was a clear, alert mind. Also, knowing the excitement they felt, the rest would balance their excitement.

They nodded in agreement and understanding. Then, we began our workout.

Those three days together in training could only be described as blissful. We spent our mornings doing exercises and drills to increase flexibility and speed, working on refining technique, discussing strategy and tactics, and engaging in light sparring. In the afternoons, we enjoyed getting to know each other: eating out together in restaurants, taking walks in parks and along the ocean. The team members formed a close bond and were easy and happy together, uplifting each other's spirits.

The team came from all over the U.S: Fred Adsher, Michael Ajay, James Butin, Roger Carpenter, Michael Warren, Albert Cheeks, Archie Ray Cole, Bobby Martin, and my best student from New York City, Joe Hayes. These names will always be with me because they formed the first Taekwondo team to travel to Korea and compete. They were groundbreakers and should be honored.

Our time was soon approaching to leave for Korea. Through some mix-up, however, our uniforms were not yet ready by the last day and we had to scramble and stencil the name of our team on our jackets and sweats ourselves. By evening, everything was settled and on the right course again, and on a beautiful, moonlit night, we flew out of L.A. for Korea. The team members seemed serious, almost reverential that night towards the experience they were about to have. It was as if the journey was just now beginning for them. For myself, too; it was my fifth trip back to Korea since coming to America eleven years ago, my last trip being almost two years ago. I remembered thinking, as the plane lifted through the clouds, that we were surely entering into a new world.

When we landed in Seoul about 15 hours later, Master Hong, Vice President of the Korean Taekwondo Association, met us at the airport and arranged our transportation to a downtown hotel where the teams in the championship were staying. Master Hong looked stylish in a blue business suit, wearing a Korean Taekwondo Association pin on his lapel. He was in high spirits.

After we registered at the hotel, Master Hong returned to his office. Just before he left, he turned to us.

"We are all looking forward to an exciting championship," he said. "We have planned a large celebration at the Silla Hotel afterwards. But, now, please get some rest. You must be tired after your long trip. Dinner will be at seven. Each team will have their own table, and the kitchen has prepared a special dinner for you."

We settled into our rooms and rested for a few hours. Then, at seven, we emerged and met in the large dining hall, where the teams of all the nations competing were gathered. It was truly inspiring to see martial artists from countries all over the world—Mexico, Italy, Germany, Japan, Philippines, Taiwan, Senegal, Ivory Coast—faces of all different races and cultures gathered together for a common purpose. Their Korean masters were seated by their sides, and I noticed, that these masters were young men like myself who had left Korea at a young age and brought the tradition of Taekwondo to these nations. I felt very proud to be among them.

Soon, dinner was served. In honor of each nation, the hotel prepared a traditional meal from that nation. This surprised me; I had been expecting a traditional Korean meal to introduce us to Korean culture. In fact, during the flight, I had excitedly told my team about classic Korean dishes.

"You must taste the Beef Bulgo Gi while you are here," I said.

Instead, that first evening, we were served hamburger on bread with a scoop of rice on the side, fried potatoes with ketchup spiced with ginger, and a salad. The dinner was not quite American in style and not quite Korean either. To be honest, it was not that good, but it didn't seem to spoil our appetites. We ate every morsel off our plates and thanked our waiter, who proudly announced with a big smile, "tomorrow's lunch is pot chicken pie with apple sauce," not knowing he twisted the name of the dish.

During dinner, Dr. Kim made his way around to each table to personally greet the team and their coaches. His assistant then informed each coach of their daily practice schedule at the Kukkiwon, the World Taekwondo Headquarters where the championship would be held. Each nation was given about an hour during the day to practice semi-privately at the gym. A line was drawn midway in the gym cutting it in half for two teams to workout simultaneously. If more time was needed for practice, we were advised to take our team to one of the nearby parks.

The following morning a small shuttle bus met us at the hotel and brought us to Kukkiwon for our morning practice session. Along the way, we traveled down roads that I knew years ago when I lived in Seoul. Back then, these roads were small with only two lanes, some still dirt and gravel. Now, everything had changed. The road was a four-lane highway and along it were many tall, newly constructed buildings. There was so much change, and I was so unfamiliar with it all. I almost felt like a foreigner in my own country. But, the faces of the Korean people, on their way to work or school, many riding bicycles, made me feel familiar and at home again. Their faces were soft and round, like mine. These were my people; here were my roots.

For the next few days, we fell rhythmically into our routine—a morning workout, an 'American' lunch (for example, pizza), a tactic session in the afternoon, some free time for resting and sightseeing, and early to bed. In a few days, the trial matches would begin, and although the team naturally felt some nervous jitters, we felt ready.

One afternoon before the trials began, I brought the team to visit the Moo Duk Kwan Institute where I first began training. I had notified Master Hong that I would be coming, and he was pleased. I was pleasantly surprised, and somewhat relieved, to see that the one-story structure looked exactly the same as I remembered it, except for a new coat of paint. We entered the school after workout for the students had already begun. Silently, we watched. There were a group of about 40 boys, ages 9 to 16 years old, practicing their forms in unison. There was a powerful silence in the gym except for an occasional yell. Master Hong stood off to the side watching them. As I watched these young students of the martial arts, I remembered back when I was a student like them. I saw myself there many years ago doing the same forms, practicing in the same way. Then, as now, the forms were practiced over and over again in these drills until they were second nature, completely internalized. Sometimes, it became boring to repeat these forms again and again, but we did it because this was our master's instruction, even if we didn't understand the effect it had on us. Now I understand that it was not only the knowledge of the form that we were perfecting, but, in essence, ourselves. Everyday, through the repetition and drill work, we were training and focusing the mind to become sharp and precise. We were integrating our mind and body into one, and before we knew it, an inner strength developed within us like an unseen muscle. This integration and unity is the supreme achievement of a martial artist, and is at the source of all his or her strength. Whether or not I understood this back then, whether or not these young students understood, this is the course of development for a martial artist. The tradition had not changed in my lifetime, since I was a student here over 20 years ago, nor had it changed since its beginnings over 2000 years ago. And the result was always the same: after a while, the forms flowed out of you like your breath, and invincibility radiated from you like a pure light. As I was absorbed in my reverie, Master Hong spotted me and immediately interrupted the practice. He approached us.

I bowed to Master Hong and then introduced the American team to him. They bowed respectfully to Master Hong, and the young Korean students watched in awe.

"Master Chun, it is very good to see you, " he said. Then, he addressed the team wishing them, "the best luck in the competition." Master Hong introduced the team to his students. They all bowed to us, then with Master Hong's instruction continued with their practice of the forms.

We watched for about 20 minutes and then we silently left. As I was about to leave, I glanced back at Master Hong and simultaneously he turned to me and nodded his head expressing love and respect. I bowed to him and turned, returning to our bus and our trip back to our hotel.

On the bus the team was very animated and talkative. They had been inspired by the visit to my old school and to see martial artists so accomplished at that age.

"At what age did you start, Master Chun?" asked a 22-year-old black belt from Texas.

"I started under Master Hong at the age of eleven and earned my black belt three years later," I said. I paused for a moment, and considered telling them the story of my early days.

"When I began," I continued, "I started martial arts for all the wrong reasons."

"What do you mean?" another team member said. All their heads turned to listen carefully. For the remainder of the bus ride home, I told the team the story of revenge that had comprised my first six months as a martial artist.

I was happy to see the team gaining an appreciation for their art. Seeing an accomplished Korean master train his students had inspired them. However, I had noticed something that concerned me, which I kept to myself. I noticed that the students we had observed were all young and just beginners. It would have been another experience to watch older black belt students workout. I had tried to arrange it when we first arrived in Seoul, but was politely refused.

At dinner one evening, I asked Master Lee, one of the coaches of the Korean team and someone whom I had known for years, if I may observe the team.

"Ah, yes, Master Chun," he said, "we shall see if we can arrange that. You know that the Korean team doesn't train at Kukkiwon. We wouldn't want to inconvenience you."

It was not a surprise that teams trained separately, yet to train in complete seclusion at another facility was odd, I thought. It only motivated me to see them that much more. Any opportunity to view the opponent beforehand was worthwhile because it could add to your strategy. I was interested in seeing what the Korean martial artists were doing. That was another reason for viewing the students at my master's school, but I had learned nothing new observing the novices.

The trials were beginning in two days, and once they began, I would be absorbed in my students and the events of the championship. My time to observe the Korean team was running out. I had only one more day to do it.

Later that evening, as I was relaxing in my room with my assistant coaches, I was lucky to receive information from a good source regarding the place where the Korean team would be practicing the following morning. An informal invitation to attend was offered to me.

By 8:30 am the next day, I quietly entered a small martial arts institute on the outskirts of the town. Practice was already in session. I sat on a folding chair off to the side and watched the team.

It was no surprise that the team was excellent in every way. They were in excellent physical shape and executed their techniques with great precision. Each team member seemed at the height of his development and each one seemed better than the next. I watched for a while as the team went through their training, then split up for some sparring. It was all routine for a while until I noticed something different. A few of the sparring pairs were using techniques that I had never seen before. I observed more closely.

They were executing variations on traditional kicks, but such variations that would prove devastating to unsuspecting opponents. One move, for instance, was an addition on the forward kick. In the traditional move, the fighter takes a quick step forward, hops quickly on one leg and then snaps the other up for a forward blow. It is a fast and powerful frontal attack move. In the new move, the leg snapped up very high. At that point, the opponent would assume the move is completed, and might even enter to initiate a counterblow. Yet, when the leg was up, it was quickly brought down again either straight or on an angle for a hit to the face or head. It was very effective. I discovered later that this kick was called the turning ax kick by the Korean team. It was just one of a few new moves that the Korean masters and their students had developed.

Soon, I left the practice session. The expression on my face was one of complete shock. My mind was whirling. How many more new moves were the Korean team perfecting? There was no way that I, as a coach, could properly prepare my team to defend against moves that I didn't know. Even if I did, there wouldn't be enough time to train them. It took hours of drill before action and reaction became routine; however, I had to at least warn them to be prepared for surprises. It had also become very clear to me why I had not been allowed to view the team until close to the start of the championship.

I was unsure of how to inform our team about these new advances that I had seen during the Korean team's practice. The trials were beginning the next day, so that afternoon I announced to our team that we would have a special session. In an hour, everyone was assembled. No one knew why. I decided to be straightforward with my team in preparing them for what would come.

"Today, I had the opportunity to view the Korean team in practice. Of course, as I expected they were well-trained and in excellent shape. This was no surprise," I said.

The team and coaches were listening intently, unaware of what I was about to say, yet knew that something was coming.

"I must tell you that during the practice session, I saw new techniques that would be very difficult to counter because of the element of surprise," I said. Then, I briefly described what I saw that afternoon. The team seemed as shocked as I was and thankful that I had alerted them to these new techniques.

"I don't know what other new tricks the Korean team has in store for us, but be prepared for anything," I said. "That is all I can tell you. We are in the country where Taekwondo originated. Even to this day, the great dedication and research done by the martial art masters is bringing about innovations in our sport and art. You have been well trained. I am sure that you will do well."

For the remainder of the day, we rested and mentally prepared ourselves for the upcoming championship that would begin the following day.

The first day of the championship was very exciting. Martial artists from 22 nations converged in the gymnasium. The teams assembled and the athletes warmed up. Everywhere, there were warm exchanges, smiles, and greetings. The auditorium was full of life and energy. Five thousand spectators looked down into the arena where two matches would be held simultaneously. A dias at one end of the auditorium, flanked by large floral arrangements, displayed the trophies and medals that would be awarded to the first, second, and third place finishers in each of three weight divisions. On the wall behind the dias, a large Korean flag was displayed surrounded by smaller flags representing all the participating nations.

There were two days of trials during which the competitors worked their way to the final matches by a process of elimination. The first day for the U.S. Team was a good one. All of our team members who fought that day advanced to the next round. Only the U.S., Mexico, Germany, and Korea advanced without losing a match. Korea, of course, advanced easily. It was obvious that their team was superior. They performed flawlessly. However, I noticed something midway through the day that began to disturb me. The judges and referees, who were Korean and members of the Korean Tae Kwan

Do Association, seemed to favor the Korean fighters in the matches. It was not intentional, I felt. Perhaps it wasn't really favoritism, but rather that they held everyone else to the superior standards of a Korean team. Thus, if a martial artist from another country executed a blow that, in my opinion, would have clearly been a scoring hit but it didn't have the speed or precision of the Korean team, the official did not score the point.

I wanted to say something, but restrained myself. I was still feeling a bit uneasy from viewing the Korean team's practice the day before, and maybe things would even out in later matches when the better fighters would perform. However, I promised myself that if an opportunity presented itself, I would raise the issue. That evening the opportunity did arise. I had been invited to dinner with some of the Korean masters and members of the association. At dinner, the conversation soon turned to the championships.

"What do you think of the competition so far, Master Chun?" said Master Lee, whom I had met only recently.

"Well, today, I am happy. All of my team advanced to the next round," I said.

"Yes, your team is performing well, Master Chun. They look very strong," said another master.

The feeling rose in me to bring up the point about the judges, but I didn't at that moment.

"Yes, thank you," I said. "We have worked hard in our short time together. And I couldn't help notice how well prepared the Korean team is."

"You were able to watch us train one day. Is that right?" said Master Li, a master from a school in Pusan.

I nodded.

"I hope you are not upset with us that we didn't share with you some of our new techniques. I'm sure you understand that we want to hold onto some of our secrets for a while, " said Master Li.

"Of course," I said. "However, I must say that I noticed something today. The officials were a bit strict in awarding points to competitors from other nations even if hits were accurate because they were not up to the standards of what you are accustomed to."

My words came out spontaneously. I wanted to hold back, but I couldn't. I hoped that I had not offended anyone. Here I was in Korea, with masters who were my peers, and I was criticizing the officials of the championship. I could see that they were surprised, but restrained their reactions, except one.

"Who's side are you on, Master Chun?" he said, half-jokingly.

I laughed, but also in a half-joking way.

"I am the coach of the U.S. team, Master Li," I said.

Our dinner continued and ended with warm good-byes, but I felt odd. I had stood up for my team, which was right. Yet, I was a Korean national. I had seen a bias in the scoring that I believed was unintentional, and I spoke about it. I felt proud of the accomplishments of my team. I was also proud of the power and mastery of the Korean team. There seemed to be many contradictory feelings, but they all lived peacefully within me.

The following morning, I met a few family members for breakfast at a beautiful hotel near the Kukkiwon, and then together we went to the second day of the trials. It was not a great day for us; two of our team members lost their matches and were eliminated. We were now down to four. However, I did notice a change in the judging—more ease in awarding points to a hit that was certainly acceptable, but not perfection according to Korean standards.

By the afternoon of the following day, when the final matches were scheduled to begin, the Kukkiwon was filled to capacity with 5000 spectators. All eyes were focused on the single mat where each weight division would go in succession. The competitors would fight three 2-minute matches with a 30 second rest between each match. Whoever scored the most points in three matches won.

Dr. Kim was beaming with happiness that day. He was elegantly dressed in a business suit and decided to watch the competition in seats down front with many dignitaries.

Before the finals began, I huddled the four American finalists together along with the assistant coaches.

"Let's take a moment of silence," I said. "You have made it this far. I am very proud of you. You have all worked hard. Now, good luck."

I put my hand on the shoulder of Joe Hayes, who had made the finals. Then, we bowed our heads in silence, each one of us praying to our own God. The excitement and activity around us disappeared as we huddled silently in a corner of the gymnasium. We were the silent center within a storm for that moment. We broke and the finals began.

Quickly, the Korean team proved their superiority by winning the first two matches easily. The new techniques that they had worked on proved effective against unsuspecting opponents. In the second match between a

Korean and a Taiwanese, the Korean used a new move that later I learned was the turning wheel kick. In this move, a hook or wheel kick motion is combined with a spinning of the body making the kick hard to pick up and determine its point of contact. While the body is turning, the kick can go upward, straight across, or downward. The complexity of the move is very difficult to defend against, particularly if the opponent has never seen it. The Taiwanese fighter was excellent, yet no match for the Korean with superior and advanced kicking techniques.

The day went by in a similar manner for the remainder of the Korean team and the opponents from the other nations. Three out of the four Americans lost their matches, including Joe Hayes, who was perhaps the best American martial artist at that time. Joe's strengths were his great combination of speed and power, but even these qualities could not compete with the speed, execution, and complexity of the Korean martial artists. Joe placed third in the lightweight division.

Two other Americans also did well. Michael Warren and Albert Cheeks from the Washington, D.C. area, both students of the late Master Ki Hwang Kim, took second and third place respectively in the heavyweight division of the championship. Michael was particularly swift even though he was a heavyweight. He applied hop round kicks followed by quick hook kicks to get points. He was the only American to place second, our highest winner.

Overall, the Koreans won the championship easily with the U.S. team placing second. Mexico and Chinese Taipei tied for third place. I was extremely proud of our team and told them that "winning second place is the best that we could do. I am very proud of you."

That evening we rested at our hotel. The next few days before our return trip home would be spent at celebrations, shopping, and sightseeing—well-earned rewards for working hard.

At lunch the next day, we had a small team celebration and then went shopping. At that time, the American dollar in Korea was very strong. We all bought gifts for our families and friends, and had suits tailor-made for ourselves. Master Won had recommended a tailor to us who made three suits for one hundred American dollars. Not one of us could pass up that excellent bargain.

We had only one more full day in Seoul, and I wanted to make it a meaningful one for our team and the whole U.S. contingent. I decided to take everyone to the Kyung-Bok Palace, just outside of Seoul. The palace was the home of the past emperors of Korea. It was a sprawling area that could take days to explore. In the grand buildings the royal families lived, played, and executed official business. There were also numerous gardens, walkways, and ponds with magnificent arched bridges. One garden, in particular, would be our destination. It was called the Biwon, or the 'Secret' Garden.

"Why is it called the Secret Garden?" asked a team member on our way to the palace.

"Because in this garden, deep within the palace confines, the masters of Taekwondo would practice their art. It was their Do Jang," I answered.

The bus took the main road out of Seoul past the hotels and business district, through the tree-lined residential sections of Seoul, then out to more rural areas where the palace lay. When we entered the main gate, it was like entering a new city and a different period of time.

We stopped to see the main palace for a while, then found a map that would guide our way to Biwon Garden. A bridge over a lovely pond filled with lotus flowers signaled our entrance into the garden.

"Look at this bridge," said Master Hwang as we walked past shapely maple trees and approached the bridge.

The eyes of the team members grew large with wonder. The bridge was constructed of stone with intricate lattice carvings and designs. The distinguishing feature of the bridge was four larger-than-life figures standing guard on the bridge, two at each end. Each figure was a Taekwondo master executing a different form. As we approached and walked past them onto the bridge, we noticed the powerful expressions on their faces: one in deep concentration like the silent stone itself, the other in the act of exhalation of breath. Although thousands of years old, you could almost feel the breath and the power of attention emanating from the figures.

As we entered the garden, the students became hushed as if respecting the history of the place. They glanced around and took everything in: the sights, sounds, and smell of this ancient place. The garden was very large, with open spaces divided into sections by flowering bushes and trees. Here, the masters of the past passed on the tradition of Taekwondo to their worthy students.

We walked through the different sections of the garden. I could see that we all felt in awe of the garden and the tradition that it represented. For the most part, we were silent. As a group, I could feel that we were all at peace within ourselves, silently connected to the greatness and vastness of the tradition of Taekwondo, which was thousands of years old. In that moment, I remember feeling a deep inner stillness and balance, as if the feeling permeated the atmosphere of the garden. At the center of this feeling was a sense of inner bliss that was greater than any happiness I had ever known. Along with this came feelings of invincibility and immortality. Never before had I felt such a mastery of life itself, and I knew that this feeling was the goal of Taekwondo and all martial arts. It was the state of spiritual enlightenment.

In the Chinese philosophy of Taoism, which is said to be the source of the martial art's philosophy, there is a belief that there is one single unchanging principle or reality behind all changing events. Recognizing and harmonizing with this 'One' is the true way to wisdom and peace. It is the source of all invincibility and power in human life, as well as in nature.

My thoughts were broken by the excited voice of a team member's discovery.

"Who's that?" he asked, pointing to a large stone statue of a man wrapped in loosely fitting robes, holding a scroll.

The expression on his face was one of complete serenity, and his physique was not at all like the chiseled look of a martial artist, but his belly was large and round and soft like a ripe fruit.

"That's Won Kwang, the monk who it is said originated Taekwondo," said Master Kang.

"A monk originated Taekwondo?" said another student. "Why did a religious man teach fighting techniques?"

"Because in essence, training in the martial arts is not about fighting techniques, but about spiritual discipline, a spiritual way," I said.

"Won Kwang was also practical," added Master Ahn. "During the Silla Dynasty when Taekwondo was formed, Korea needed to defend itself from its numerous foes. Taekwondo emerged out of our spiritual need to maintain selfhood and dignity as a people.

"So the tradition of the martial artist in Korea is connected to the survival of the Korean people? " asked a team member.

"Yes," I said. "It simultaneously evolved into a powerful spiritual system. Won-Kwang is the source of the Taekwondo tradition and he is also the goal."

"What is the goal of our studies, Master Chun? Surely, it is more than just achieving a black belt," asked a team member.

"Yes, there is more. The goal is enlightenment," I said.

"And what is enlightenment?" asked another team member.

"Enlightenment is a mastery of life. It means overcoming all inner obstacles and fears. It is invincibility, knowledge, and peace. It is fulfilling your dreams and aspirations. It is forever growing into a more perfect, loving, contented, humble, successful human being. And it is sharing this experience with others who are traveling down that same path with you," I said.

"And this is our path," said Master Ahn.

"Yes, we are all traveling down it together," said another team member.

"Yes, this is our way—our 'Do'," I said.

Soon, we were out of the Biwon Garden and on our way home, but our discussion about the wholeness and tradition of our martial art continued throughout the entire day.

As I had predicted months ago, before coming to Korea with the American team, this journey to the birthplace of our tradition would be a lasting memory for all of us. That intuition proved to be correct.

That evening, a grand celebration for all the martial artists who participated in the championships was held in an elegant ballroom at the luxurious Silla Hotel. Everyone was relaxed and happy. There was interesting conversation and much laughter. There were many speeches and toasts and Dr. Kim presented many awards and honors. I remember at one point during his talk, he told us, "Fulfill your destinies as martial artists. Go out to every corner of the world and radiate the light of consciousness that is alive within a master of the martial arts. This will be good for you, for all those around you, and for the world as a whole."

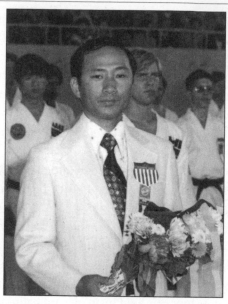

Richard Chun, head coach of the U.S.A. team to the first World Taekwondo Championship, Seoul, Korea, 1973, in which the U.S.A. team won second place.

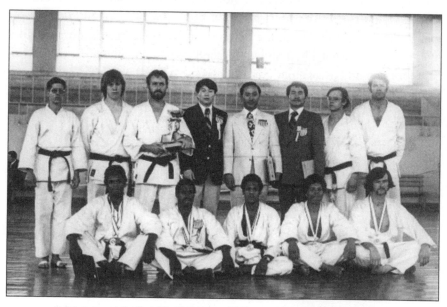

U.S.A. team at the first World Taekwondo Championship, Seoul Korea, 1973.

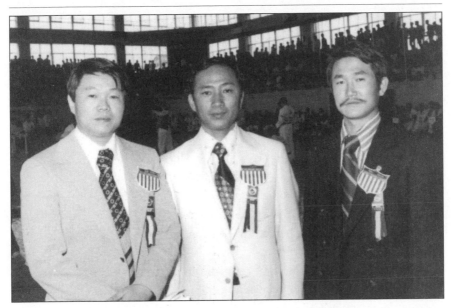

Richard Chun, Head Coach (center); Il Hoi Kim, Assistant Coach (left); Dae Hyun Kim, Assistant Coach (right); at the first World Taekwondo Championship, Seoul Korea, 1973.

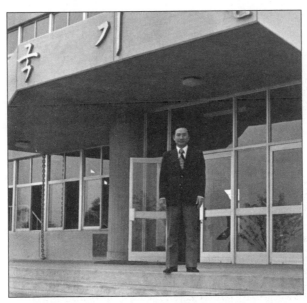

Richard Chun, Special Assistant to the President of the World Taekwondo Federation, Dr. Un Yong Kim, in front of Kukkiwon (World Taekwondo Center), where the first World Taekwondo Championship was held, 1973.

CHAPTER 9

The Missing Piece

Twenty-two students, ranging from 10 to 19 years in age, lined up before me to demonstrate their skills. They bowed quickly at the command of their master, Kae Jun. It was a disorganized bow, not at all in unison, but more like the out-of-step march of an undisciplined army troop. I glanced over to Kae Bae Jun and smiled. He returned my acknowledgement with a gentle nod of his head.

Master Jun was a young, but respected, Korean black belt with a bushy head of black hair, seemingly always unkempt. He was short and muscular and had a particularly small nose. I had sponsored Master Jun to live in the United States. In Korea, he was a student of Master Jae Chun from the city of Kwang Joo, but all his life he dreamed of coming to the United States. In Korea, Kae Jun was an accomplished martial artist; he taught military personnel at the Army base and he was also a martial arts instructor at the Police Academy in Seoul. In the late 1960's, he was hired to be on the team of personal security guards protecting the Prime Minister of Korea, who was then the most powerful commander in the military junta. During that time, he met Dr. Kim who worked closely with the Prime Minister as his right-hand man. One day, Kae Jun mentioned to Dr. Kim that he was interested in moving to the United States and asked if he had contacts there. Of course, Dr. Kim told him about me. In 1969, I accepted Kae Jun as my assistant instructor and arranged for his move to New York.

Kae Jun stayed with me a little over a year, sharing space in my apartment. A few years younger than I with some common experiences growing up in Korea, we quickly became friends. Once here, he immediately immersed himself in American culture and language. He was a quick learner and wanted to absorb American customs as quickly as possible so he could behave and relate to the American people on their own terms. As a martial art instructor in my school, we also worked together on designing new teaching methods for the American martial art student.

I had learned during my years here that teaching American students was different from teaching Korean students. The American student seemed to need more explanation than the Korean. An obvious reason for this was that Taekwondo was not part of the American cultural landscape, and therefore my students were unfamiliar with it. Another reason, I believe, was an innate cultural difference in the way of thinking between the Korean and American people. Americans seemed to expect things faster. For example, in Korea, a martial art master instructs and demonstrates a technique to his students. After making corrections and being sure that his students have learned the basics of the technique, the students drill that technique over and over again until the move becomes second nature. This was the routine in almost every martial arts school. This was the procedure for learning in general. The student understood that they would not progress to the next level until the previous one had been mastered. On the other hand, I noticed that in the U. S., American students naturally enjoyed learning a new technique and how to execute it. They did practice the technique diligently, but they soon became bored with the drill work, and wanted to go on to a different technique before perfecting the previous one. From the Korean perspective, they seemed to lack the patience to work single-mindedly on one thing. They would rather gather more and more information even before they might be ready for it. I noticed this was the mentality of the American student, and it was different from the Korean. Now, I am not criticizing the American student's dedication to their art, which I observed was strong and full of feeling and energy. I believe strongly in the freedom and abundance that the American society offers, but the value of patience in developing one's art was not as ingrained in them as I had been accustomed to seeing in young Korean martial art students.

Master Jun also noticed this difference when he first came to assist me at my school. For the six months that he stayed with me in New York, we talked about this difference often and worked at adjusting our teaching methods to better fit the American student all while maintaining the integrity of our tradition. It was a delicate balance. During that time, I gained a fine appreciation of Master Jun; he was an excellent martial artist and an enterprising and independent young man. I was not surprised, therefore, that when an opportunity arose for Master Jun to work with a former black belt of mine, Carlos Rivera, to set up a school in Youngstown, Ohio, he grabbed it.

Carlos had moved to Youngstown with his wife three years ago to take a job there, but he had always wanted to start a school of his own. Finally, he had saved and earned enough money to do so. Kae Jun moved to Ohio to assist Carlos. In one short year, they had built a good business together and they invited me to spend a weekend there to observe their students and teach them new techniques. It was a pleasure for me to do so. It had been my habit during this time, as my name and reputation as a martial artist grew, to visit schools across the country for a few days at a time.

Their school in Youngstown was situated in a large office building in the center of the town. It was very well equipped for a martial arts school in a small town with hanging punching bags, large mirrors, and a brand new wooden floor. The students were neatly dressed in their starched white doboks with the emblem of *Youngstown Martial Arts School* sewn on their uniforms over their chest. In many ways, the school reminded me of the numerous other schools that I had visited during the year. They were popping up in many small towns and cities all over the U.S. and they were all the same—modest in scale and numbers teaching a blend of techniques and styles all under the generic name of "karate."

Master Jun instructed his students to begin the demonstration. The students went through a series of forms for about 30 minutes. They threw their bodies around executing kicks and punches, interspersed with hand movements, blocking techniques, and even rolls. I saw Taekwondo, Hopkido, Jujitsu, Kung-Fu, Karate and other martial arts styles thrown together into one melting pot, creating quite a unique blend.

One thing I have learned about myself over the years as a martial artist is that I am a purist. I had been taught in the pure tradition of Taekwondo, without the mixture of other styles. I felt fortunate to have had this type of training, because I was able to delve deeply into the essence of Taekwondo. In the United States, however, there was a blending taking place within the schools. This approach had its pros and cons. The blending of styles brought out the strengths of each system, such as the falling techniques of Judo, the hand techniques of Jujitsu, or the breaking holds of Aikido and Hopkido. Too much mixing, however, created confusion in the mind of the student and a lack of stability and connection to one tradition and Master.

In my own school, I focused on Taekwondo. The demand and numbers in a city the size of New York were there. However, in smaller towns and cities martial art schools were forced to blend many styles in order to survive. They called it self-defense, karate or jujitsu, which was the most recognizable name, to attract students. This was the type of school that my former student and Kae Jun established in Youngstown.

Frankly though, it wasn't so much the confused blending of styles that disappointed me, but rather the actual performance of the forms. The execution was unsophisticated, oversimplified, and not very precise. In fact, the students were sloppy in their performance. They did not seem to have a concept of mastering the form, but instead just performed for the fun of it. I saw that the students did not understand the seriousness of their study of the martial arts.

I wanted to speak out, but I held back my disappointment, not exactly sure of how to respond at that moment. When the students finished their performance, I stood up and bowed in their direction. The next day, I was to lead the workout. This was when I would try to correct what I saw. I would also speak to Kae Jun and Carlos when the opportunity arose.

After the workout, I rested for a while in my room at Carlos' house. Then Carlos, Kae Jun, and I spent an informal evening at a local restaurant talking about old times and enjoying each other's company. Although the opportunity did arise to raise the issues of what I had seen that day, I let the matter pass. It didn't seem like the right time to bring up this business matter. I would talk to them about it tomorrow. That night, we were simply out for fun and enjoyment.

The following morning we met bright and early with the students for a workout. They were gathered together, all eager and ready. When they saw me in my doboks, they approached me with numerous questions.

"What new kicks are we going to learn today, Master Chun?"

"Did you like our performance yesterday?"

"Are we going to spar today, Master Chun?"

I surprised them with my response.

"Today, we are not going to learn new techniques," I said.

There was a hush and a feeling of anticipation in the air.

"Instead," I continued, "we are going to refine the ones we already know."

I saw by their unenthusiastic response that my plan had disappointed them, and Kae Jun, noticing their reaction, was embarrassed.

He clapped his hands a few times to get their attention.

"Now line up and get prepared for instruction," he said. "We are very fortunate to have Master Chun with us this weekend."

They lined up reluctantly. I approached the students.

"Yesterday, I noticed that when many of you executed the round kick, your weight was too far forward. This will throw your balance off," I said.

I took a step toward them.

"Your center of gravity should be here," I said, pointing to my stomach. "When your balance is off, your speed will slow down, and the precision and power of the technique will be missing."

The students were listening carefully.

"Here, watch me," I said.

I walked to the center of the gym floor and stood there for a few seconds. Then, I bowed to them to illustrate that we were all engaged not only in the practice of a technique, but actually part of a tradition and working on mastery of the self. No words were necessary, the action would speak for itself. I executed the technique of a round kick perfectly for them.

"Wow," I heard some of the students say. "That was great."

"Now back into your lines," I said. "Before we learn new kicking techniques, you must practice this one many times."

Kae Jun and Carlos were off to the side of the floor watching with smiles on their faces.

"You must practice this kick at least 50 times a day for the next two weeks. It will take you that long before you master it," I said.

"50 times," one student exclaimed.

"What about sparring?" said another.

"Before we spar don't you think it is important that we master the techniques we are going to use?" I inquired. I put it in question form because I wanted to understand their thinking.

"I think we know it enough, Master Chun," said one student. "I can do it in the tournament two weeks from now."

"Ah, yes, the tournament coming up. How many of you are in the tournament?" I said.

Every hand went high into the air. Pointing to one student, I asked how many trophies he had won.

"Three," he answered proudly.

"Very good," I said. "Now, let's practice the round kick—50 times."

I felt their disappointment rise again.

We worked on the round kick for another 15 or 20 minutes, amidst some groaning as if I were torturing them, but we nevertheless continued. I ended the morning session with some light sparring. The practice was a revelation to me, and after all the students left and only Carlos and Kae Jun were left, we sat down for a talk. Jun apologized for the verbal outbursts of the student's, which he thought showed disrespect to the master.

"Thank you, Master Jun," I said. "I appreciate that, but what concerns me even more is what I saw this morning not only in your school, but in many schools across the country."

"What, Master Chun?" said Carlos.

"It is the attitude of the students," I said. "They are here only for the sport of it—to quickly learn some punches and kicks for competition and trophies."

Carlos and Kae Jun hung their heads in disappointment and shame.

"It is not your fault. Don't feel bad," I said. "As I said, I have seen this attitude all over the country ... and even in my school."

They were surprised to hear that.

"Yes, even in my own school. I am always coming across students who are there just because they want to win some medals or trophies to put up on their shelves at home. Now, there is nothing wrong with medals or trophies as long as it doesn't become the only reason for training. Most of the time these students do not last long, once they see the hard work it takes to win a few medals or trophies."

"What do you do in this situation, Master Chun?" said Carlos.

"Well, once a young student of mine lost out on winning a trophy at a tournament. He was very upset, almost in tears. I was torn as to how I should approach him. I knew his feelings were hurt and delicate at the moment, but I also knew that the trophy was all he cared about. He was not thinking about the experience and growth in his training," I said.

I picked up a small trophy that was on a desk in their office.

"I went over to the boy with a trophy like the one he would have won. I congratulated him on his performance and asked him to look at and feel the trophy. What is it made of?" I asked him.

He looked puzzled, but did what I asked him. He reached out and touched the trophy.

"It is made of wood and metal," he said.

"That's right, " I said. "Two very strong substances. It would be hard to break this in half, wouldn't it?" I asked him."

He nodded.

"Imagine you becoming that strong," I said.

He looked amazed and also confused.

"Your training is not all about winning trophies," I said. "It is about becoming as strong as metal and wood. Then, no one can break you. You become like a trophy within yourself. You know who you are, everywhere and at anytime. A real trophy you leave on a shelf, but you carry your inner strength wherever you go. You can become as strong as metal and as sturdy as wood. This is what you need to develop. This is what your training in the martial arts is all about. Keep your mind on that and, before you know it, you will have more trophies than you ever imagined. But, none will be as important as what you develop within."

Carlos and Kae Jun smiled.

"What ever happened to that student?" Carlos said.

"He became one of my best black belts," I said.

"But back to our problem at hand," I continued. "It seems to me that many students today are unaware of this deeper meaning in the martial arts. They do not see something greater than just physical skill. We must take the blame partially for this."

"Yes, Master Chun, you are right," said Kae Jun. "We know this, but you also know the problems facing us. If we make their training too hard and rigid, they will quit. If they quit, our numbers will fall, and if our numbers fall, then we will be forced to close the school."

"I am aware of this," I said, "but I am still concerned that the students are not being taught in the correct way. It is a serious dilemma."

"Tomorrow, before you leave, please talk to the students," said Carlos. "See if they will listen to you. "

I agreed.

After our conversation, I took a walk while Carlos and Kae Jun cleaned the gym and prepared it for our workout and meeting tomorrow. I understood the situation that they were in. Carlos and Kae Jun were both trained in the tradition of Taekwondo, yet felt that they had to modify and blend this tradition with other styles, watering it down so that it was easier for students to learn. It was a business decision, and their number one priority was to stay in business. Yet, to do so, much of the strength in the martial art was being diluted, not to mention the loss of the link to the philosophical tradition.

In New York, Kae Jun and I modified our teaching style to adjust to the American student. Maybe that first step was one step too far off the path of our tradition because one step always led to another. Before you knew it, too much would have been sacrificed. I felt frustrated and disturbed about what I saw. My experience in Youngstown was not different from what I saw all over the U.S., and even with some of my own students, at first.

The martial arts were certainly gaining popularity. There was no doubt about it. It was a decade of tremendous growth in the U.S. There were masters creating black belts every day and many of these black belts were opening schools in cities and towns all over the country. The fact remained that, in my view, the essence of the art was being lost. It was slowly eroding due to overwhelming business concerns and compromises. The more I thought about it, the more I couldn't bear to have it that way.

I decided that something had to be done. But what? What could one person do against this growing trend? The only answer that came to me was try to set right what was wrong wherever I saw it. No matter how small a point it seemed. That was all I could do, and that is what I would do. The next afternoon I would be leaving, but in the morning I was scheduled to meet the students for a final workout. I would start my crusade to put the essence of Taekwondo back into the art. That evening after dinner with Carlos and his wife, I rested in my room and tried to figure out how to accomplish this goal. I didn't have much luck and eventually decided to retire to bed.

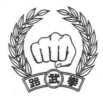

MOO DUK KWAN EMBLEM

Before drifting off to sleep that evening, I tossed and turned for a while. My mind was over-active, thinking about what I would say to the students the next morning, trying to figure out how I could correct this lack of understanding of the art of Taekwondo in schools everywhere. How could I fill in the missing piece? Wherever I turned I came up empty. Then something extraordinary happened. Out of nowhere, the symbol of the Moo Duk Kwan Institute—a fist surrounded by laurel leaves—flashed across my mind's eye. I saw every detail of the emblem as clearly as if I were looking upon it on paper.

I began to think of its meaning. The fourteen laurel leaves on each side represented the fourteen states in Korea and the advancement of peace; the three seeds on the laurel branches represented the "three thousand Li," the distance of the length of Korea; the six seeds in total represented the six continents of the world; the fist represented Taekwondo and its values of justice and righteousness; the Korean character in the center meant Moo Duk Kwan; the character on the left meant Tae (fist) and the character on the right meant Kwon (foot); the deep blue color of the emblem represented the three oceans and black belts. The emblem as a whole symbolized the spreading of the martial arts with its objectives of peace and human advancement throughout the entire world. This was the tradition to which I belonged and to which I was now dedicating my work.

This vision reminded me that the tradition of Taekwondo was too rich and complete to sacrifice and compromise. I didn't know how I would do it, but I was sure that I had to remain firm and resolute in maintaining the purity of the martial arts. If I always remained true to its heart and essence, I believed all else would follow.

The following morning, we all assembled again for our workout. I put the students through a long stretching and warm-up session. Then, we drilled over and over again a few of the moves that they had learned. Midway through the morning, I stopped the workout and gathered the students together. At this point, I would normally spend some time instructing the students in their forms, either correcting their technique or adding new ones. This morning, however, was different. I began with a question.

"Do any of you know where the tradition of the martial arts began?" I said.

"In Japan," answered a student.

"In China," another student called out.

"Korea," answered another.

"Yes, yes, you are all right. The martial arts began in Asia. Each country created their own unique form of martial art," I said.

The students became animated, wanting to show off their knowledge.

"Why do you think these styles of martial art began? What was its purpose?" I questioned.

"For self-defense."

"To protect the country."

"To fight enemies," were some of the answers of the students.

"Again, you are right, but only partially right. It is true the martial arts originated as a weapon or means of self-defense against outside invaders and foes. However, the martial arts also existed as a means for achieving growth and harmony in one's individual life."

"Really?" said a student.

"How?" asked another.

"Let me answer that question by asking you another question. What are the names of some of these styles of martial arts, do you know?" I asked.

Almost in unison, they all blurted out answers.

"Taekwondo," said one student.

"Kung-Fu," said another.

"Aikido."

"Karate," I heard.

"Judo."

"Yes, yes, very good," I said.

By now, each student felt very much a part of the lesson, listening intently for what would come next.

"Do any of you know what the *Do* means in Taekwondo or Judo?" I asked.

They were stumped by this question. No one knew the answer.

"We see this word often in the names of certain styles of martial art, such as Aikido, Hapkido, Judo" I said, emphasizing the last syllable in each case.

"The word *Do* in the martial arts means *the way*," I said.

I looked carefully at the student's faces. They looked puzzled.

"Why do you think it is called *the way?*" I said.

Again, there was no answer.

"It is called the way because to become a martial artist you must place yourself—body and mind—on a path. Like a path in the forest or in a field. When you follow a path, you know you will eventually reach the end. There is a destination. But, you also know that to reach your destination, you cannot deviate from that path, or else you may become lost. Becoming a martial artist is also like being on a path, but it is a path of complete development of body, mind, and spirit. That path is our journey, our way, our 'Do.' This process takes time, and it happens only through hard work, discipline, and respect for ourselves, our teacher, and our tradition."

The students sat around me. I wondered whether they were really listening, or just hearing my words.

"You must be serious on your path to becoming a martial artist. Make it your goal to become a true martial *artist*," I said, emphasizing the word artist. I continued.

"A martial artist is not someone who knows a few punches and kicks, or someone who has won a few trophies in a competition. Anyone can do that. That is not the destination of a martial artist on his way. And that is not what you will take with you out into the world after your practice sessions. The essence of being a martial artist is much greater than that, a benefit that will be with you wherever you go and whatever you do."

"What is that, Master Chun?" asked one student.

"When you succeed in becoming a martial artist, you will discover a great strength within you. This strength in body, mind, and spirit will help you overcome any obstacles in life, and help you achieve any goal. There will be nothing that can stand in your way. Imagine that."

The students were all listening with complete attention. I really couldn't tell if the students were absorbing this message or even ready to comprehend it, but I felt that I had to say those words. Even if I planted the seed for one martial artist that day, I would consider it a success.

"What rank are you?" I asked, looking at one student.

"High yellow," he responded.

"And you?" I said, looking at another.

"Green," he said.

"And you," I continued, looking to another.

"Red."

"Why are their different color belts?" I asked. "Do you know?"

"To show our progress," called out a student.

"That is right," I said. "But, what is the significance of the different colors?"

No one answered.

"When you begin your training in the martial arts you start with a white belt. Right?" I said.

They all nodded.

"White signifies purity and innocence. You are new on the path and hardly know anything. As you progress with time your white belt becomes more and more used or soiled and it becomes darker. It takes on a deeper and deeper color until it is no longer white, but black. That is why we progress through different color belts, each getting darker in color, until we arrive at the black belt."

"Oh," a few students said as if they had been woken up.

"How long does it take to become a black belt, Master Chun?" asked a student.

"That depends on how hard the student works," I said. "It could take many years."

"How long did it take you, Master Chun?" asked a student.

"It took me three years of dedicated training. Everyday ... in the best school in Korea," I said.

"Wow," said another student.

"How long does it take to become a martial artist, Master Chun?" asked someone. I was pleased with this question since it showed that he was truly listening.

"I am still becoming one," I said and everyone burst out in laughter, particularly Carlos and Kae Jun. However, they also knew that I was serious in my remark.

"The time doesn't matter. Just work hard and be patient, and maybe, one day, one of you will even surpass my rank," I said.

"Surpass your rank," exclaimed a student in the back, who until this time had sat quietly and not said a single word.

"Yes — one of the happiest moments in a master's life is to see his students become better than himself. Then, he knows that he has truly been a master."

I paused. There was a silence in the atmosphere. Not an empty silence, but a rich one, as if everyone was absorbing what we had just talked about. I felt I had talked enough.

"Alright, everyone back in line. Let's continue to practice our techniques. We were working on the round kick," I said.

The students hopped up like ready soldiers into their practice lines. With great enthusiasm, they began their practice again under the supervision of their masters Kae Jun and Carlos. During the practice, I saw a focus that I hadn't seen before in these students, and I felt that my little lesson on philosophy had an impact. It seemed like I had taken the correct step with them that morning, and I pledged to do this more often with all students wherever I would meet them. This was the beginning of my mission to see that the art of Taekwondo is never overshadowed by the sport.

The session ended, and soon I was on a plane heading back to New York. During the trip home, every event of the weekend passed through my mind many times until I eventually became drowsy and drifted off to sleep. Then, before I knew it, the plane had touched down and I was on my way back to my school and into my routine here in New York. The days soon began to flow by quickly.

A few weeks later, I spoke to Master Jun on the telephone. He expressed a great appreciation for my visit and told me that the students seemed more motivated since then.

"Only time will tell if they can maintain it," I said.

"You are right, Master Chun, but you have also motivated Carlos and myself," said Jun. "We will keep our students motivated."

"Yes, that is our work," I said.

When I said that phrase, a light went on in my head.

How true. It is up to us, the masters and instructors across the country to maintain the purity of our traditions. Only through that purity will Taekwondo keep its immense and glorious power throughout the ages. This was the thought I had. It was a simple thought but one that would eventually grow into the establishment of the United States Taekwondo Association ten years later.

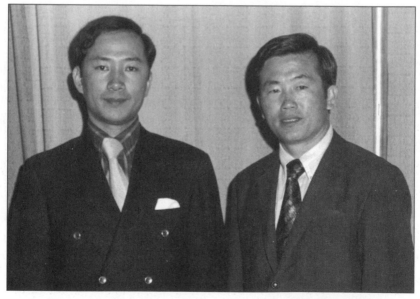

Richard Chun (left) and Grandmaster Kae Bae Chun, in Youngstown, Ohio.

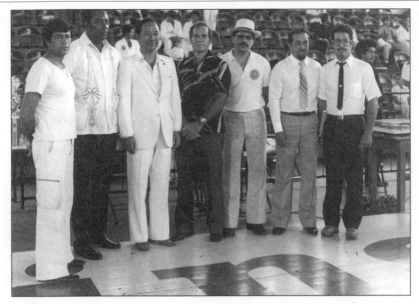

Richard Chun (third from left), Special Assistant to the President of the World Taekwondo Federation at the Caribbean Taekwondo Championship, Ponce, Puerto Rico, 1980.

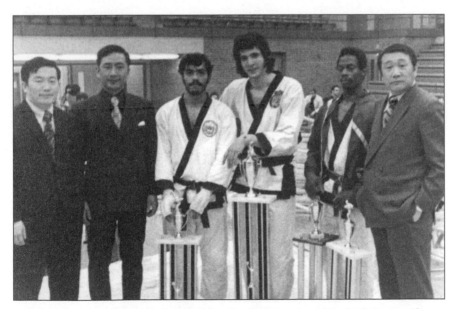

At Grandmaster Ki Whang Kim's (right) Tang Soo Do Tournament, Maryland, Kae Bae Chun (left), Richard Chun, (second from left).

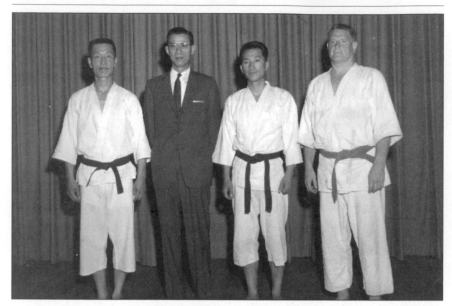

After Taekwondo demonstrations at the United Nations for the diplomats. Left to right; Grandmaster Duk Sung Son, Korean ambassador Chang Young Lim, Richard Chun, Dr. Clark, 1964.

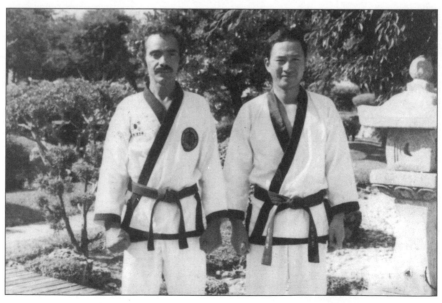

Richard Chun with his senior student and senior master instructor, Jimmy Diaz, Miami, Florida, 1967.

CHAPTER 10

Koryo Poomse

All day, a family-like atmosphere permeated the gymnasium at the Dalton School on the Upper East Side of Manhattan. On that day—May 22, 1993—I celebrated my thirty-first year as an instructor in the martial arts in the United States. To add some excitement to the celebration, I organized an inter-school tournament called "The United States Invitational Taekwondo Championships."

The championship was for members only. Students of my school, The Richard Chun Taekwondo Center, (located a block away from the gymnasium), as well as students from affiliated branches in the New York Metropolitan area and several United States Taekwondo Association schools were invited. Unlike an open tournament where anyone could enter and participate, our championship consisted of martial artists associated with my schools only, creating a warm, family environment.

Several hundred trophies, medals, and awards were presented to participants competing in forms, breaking, and free sparring. The competitions went smoothly with many outstanding performances by male and female, young and old. I was proud to see so many martial artists, many of whom had earned their belts from instructors that I had trained, performing well and also having fun. After the contests and the presentation of awards, the official ceremonies began. I started it off by introducing the attending celebrities and head instructors, and thanking all the participants and guests for attending. Then, it was my turn to be honored.

Two of my head instructors, who had been with me for many years, presented me with a large bronze trophy of a Taekwondo kicking figure. On the solid wood base beneath the figure a brass plaque read "To Grandmaster Richard Chun and Thirty-One Years of Devoted Service to Teaching Taekwondo." It is a beautiful trophy that I proudly display in the reception area of my school. After the presentation of the trophy, the youngest members of my school, the 13 year olds, presented me with a bouquet of flowers.

I was about to step in front of the microphone to give my thanks when suddenly my son and daughter emerged from a side entrance carrying a large cake covered with vanilla frosting and decorated with colorful swirls.

"What's this?" I exclaimed.

"Surprise! Happy birthday!" they said as the entire gymnasium erupted in cheers and applause.

On the cake it read, "Thirty-One years of devoted service. Fifty-eight years of good life. Happy Birthday, Grandmaster Richard Chun."

I was touched to the core of my being, and utterly surprised. I had no idea that they had organized a surprise birthday celebration to coincide with the event. The fact that my birthday had passed three months ago really didn't matter that much.

"Happy birthday," said members of the Black Belt Club who stepped up to me.

"How long have you all been planning this?" I said.

"We did a good job at keeping it a secret, didn't we?" said the black belt members.

My wife, Kwang, approached me.

"Here's a birthday wish from Dr. Kim," she said handing me a greeting card. Dr. Kim was in Korea. "He couldn't be here, but wanted to send his greetings. However, we do have another presentation and a very special guest here to honor you on your thirty first anniversary."

"Who's that?" I said.

Kwang approached the microphone and spoke softly to the assembly.

"Today, to help us celebrate this occasion, we have a special guest, one whom you all know. I would like to introduce to you the next Mayor of New York City, Mr. Rudolph Giuliani."

I think I let out a gasp in surprise and honor.

At the time of the anniversary, the soon-to-be Mayor Giuliani was in the midst of his mayoral campaign, which of course, he won that fall. His son, Andrew, had been a student of mine at the time and had progressed to green belt. I was very happy that Mayor Giuliani was able to be there. He began his speech.

"Thank you very much, Mrs. Chun, all the students of the Richard Chun Taekwondo Center and its affiliated branches, and all the guests present here today."

Everyone clapped. By now, I was starting to feel a bit embarrassed by all the attention. The Mayor continued.

"We are here on this auspicious occasion to honor Grandmaster Richard Chun who has spent more than half his life—31 years in the United States—as an instructor in the martial arts. I first met Dr. Chun last year when my son began studying under him. Immediately, I was impressed by his knowledge and dedication. It is clear upon meeting him and getting to know him that Dr. Chun is the embodiment of the martial art tradition. He radiates an inner strength and self-confidence that is rare in the world today. Almost sixty, he is healthy and fit, and he has the fearlessness of one trained in the martial arts. Yet, above all this, Dr. Chun exudes an air of serenity and peace around him."

The gymnasium was perfectly quiet; you could have heard a pin drop. The audience was silent and still, listening to the words of the Mayor. I was standing beside him, not used to all the attention, my heart beating a mile a minute, pounding like a freight train.

"And for the past 30 years, Dr. Chun has tirelessly devoted his time teaching the martial arts through his center here in New York City. By teaching our youth to pursue physical, mental, and spiritual excellence through the martial arts, Dr. Chun is providing an invaluable service to this community and city."

Everyone stood and clapped, and the clapping went on for about 5 minutes.

The celebration continued with my senior black belt teaching assistant, representing all the black belts present, stepped up to the podium.

"I would like to take a moment to list some of Dr. Chun's lifetime achievements," he said. Again, the audience became silent. As I listened, it was a proud moment for me.

"Dr. Chun is a 9th Dan Grandmaster of Taekwondo, starting his studies at age 11 in his boyhood town of Seoul, Korea. Of the more than 50 years practicing Taekwondo, Dr. Chun has been teaching it to others for 45 years. He has owned and operated a school—now on 86th Street—since 1962, training thousands of students, many of whom have gone on to open schools of their own and are here today."

"Dr. Chun," he continued, "is also the Founder and President of the United States Taekwondo Association, promoting the sport and art of Taekwondo. Besides all these achievements, Dr. Chun has found the time to earn an M.B.A. in Marketing, and a Ph.D. in Education. He is an astute businessman and a dedicated teacher. In addition, being a true humanitarian at heart, Dr. Chun is an active member of the Lions Clubs International. And finally, Dr. Chun is a devoted family man with a lovely wife and two children. Before we ask him to say a few words to you, we want to present him with this gift on behalf of all his black belt students, past and present."

Then, to add to the surprises of the day, two of my most devoted head instructors appeared carrying a large object draped in cloth. I couldn't imagine what was underneath. Speaking to the crowd, they said that this gift was in appreciation for the years of hard work and service given tirelessly to his students. As they concluded, they unveiled the object, revealing a poster-size photo of myself performing the first position of the Koryo Poomse form. It was a powerful image. Everyone in the gymnasium cheered.

All that could be seen in the photo was my head, shoulders, arms, and hands. Koryo Poomse is a black belt form where the opening position is your hands out in front of you about face level. The hands are open, palms facing outward, and the arms are extended, but not fully. There is no movement in the first position, just perfect stillness and poise. It is a very important and fundamental position and sets the tone for the entire form.

The actual name of the form, Koryo Poomse, literally means 'form of Korea.' The name Korea comes from the word Ko-Ryo, the name of the ancient dynasty that ruled between the years 918 to 1392. The people of the Ko-Ryo dynasty were known for their strong convictions and will. They consistently resisted numerous attacks from the Mongolians and thus became known for their indomitable spirit, wisdom, and strength.

The form as a whole expresses the way to cultivate strength with the precision and firm conviction in every motion, demonstrating confidence and strong will. The ready (Junbi) position, called Mom Tong Milgi means 'pushing a heavy barrel,' because it looks as if you are pushing a very heavy object like a barrel. It is the physical expression of firmness and resoluteness, as well as silence. It symbolizes, in essence, the goal of the martial artist, which is stillness or silence of being arising out of one's sense of invincibility and mastery of one self. It is no surprise that the final position of the Koryo Poomse form is also the same as the opening ready position. Stillness, silence, and resoluteness are the beginning and ending point.

After I was presented with the photo, it was my turn to speak. I felt honored and humbled by all the attention. First, I thanked the Mayor for his presence and his words. I thanked everyone for attending the tournament and celebration, and then I spoke on a more serious note.

"Standing in front of this photo which begins the form called Koryo Poomse, I am reminded of the goal of the martial artist. That goal is *not* to win as many tournaments as you can, although participating in tournaments is fun and part of a martial artist's life. You must always remember that the martial arts are not just a sport, but also an art. You play a sport—however you live the martial arts."

Everyone looked at me, ready to soak up what I was about to say.

"As a martial artist, you are a warrior, and as a warrior, you carry great responsibility and honor. Your first and foremost obligation is to yourself—to strive to live a life of peace and good character. You accomplish this through hard work and training as a fighter. As you grow in mastery of the arts of combat, you will find that you are simultaneously growing in mastery of your self, and you will also find that you are naturally becoming more humble in life," I said, looking at the hundreds of faces who had crowded the gymnasium. I continued.

"A martial artist knows humility—a humility that arises out of inner peace in their life. You can understand this experience by observing a simple rice plant. When the rice is fully matured, the stalk leans forward as if bowing down. Likewise, when a martial artist is fully matured, he or she has gained self-knowledge and inner strength. You know who you are, therefore, there is no need to boast or show off. This state of life creates humility, silence, and peace within oneself."

I felt everyone concentrating on my words.

"What comes out of this humbleness, interestingly, is the firm desire to teach and be a leader for others who are on a similar path. Because of this I opened my school and established branch schools through my black belts. Yet, I think the one accomplishment that I am most proud of is the establishment of the U.S. Taekwondo Association. Through this association I lead others on the path to achieve their goal as a martial artist, and not just as a sportsman."

Everyone, particularly my black belt students and instructors, stood up and clapped. I concluded my speech and the celebration, and the day resumed with casual socializing. It was very enjoyable with an easy feeling, yet the thought about the development and history of the U. S. Taekwondo Association remained on my mind for a long while.

I had started the U.S. Taekwondo Association twelve years earlier out of a need to promote Taekwondo as an art as well as a sport. After spending numerous years traveling around the country, visiting martial arts centers, I came to the conclusion that the art and philosophy of Taekwondo was being lost. I decided to establish the association to promote its deeper and more holistic meaning to all. More than just a sport where one accumulates trophies and ribbons, Taekwondo is a way of life that guides one towards perfection and enlightenment in life.

For years, wherever I traveled, I began to promote this *art to* teachers and students. Out of it grew the U.S. Taekwondo Association. When I established the association, members quickly joined. We created national standards for practice and competition, provided training, testing, and accreditation for individuals and schools, and sponsored seminars and tournaments. Through the association, we assisted students, instructors, and masters towards higher levels of accomplishment. On a practical level, we provided reading material and newsletters, offered discounts on martial art merchandise, and even group insurance through the association. I was very proud to create this organization in the United States and watch it grow.

Towards the end of the day as the guests began to leave and the number of competitors had thinned out, I found myself relaxing among a group of instructors and black belt students. They were telling funny stories about training, joking, and laughing together. This was a bit out of the ordinary for me because as their teacher, I was accustomed to keeping a little distance between myself and my students socially in order to keep the student-teacher relationship intact. However, today was a very special day and I let my guard down a bit. At one point during our conversation, an assistant instructor asked me to talk more about why I felt that the creation of the association was my greatest accomplishment. I paused for a second.

"Do you recall when I spoke to the group about the meaning of Koryo Poomse?" I asked.

They all nodded.

"Well, there is another meaning in that form that I didn't talk about," I said.

"What is it, Grandmaster Chun?" a black belt student said.

"The hands up and extended symbolize moving something very heavy," I said.

"Yes," said some students waiting for the answer. They knew that already.

"Moving something very heavy, yes, but maybe even, the impossible. Koryo Poomse symbolizes overcoming any obstacle, even a seemingly impossible one. My desire to see that Taekwondo remains a complete art and not just a sport for sport's sake seemed impossible to me years ago. I didn't know how to change the situation, and I wondered what one man could do. The establishment of the association was my way to move the impossible."

"As you said before, Master Chun, the goal of a martial artist is to be a leader through one's life," said an instructor.

"That's right," I said.

"Did you learn all this in the dojang, Grandmaster Chun?" asked another instructor.

"Yes, I did. The dojang as you know is not just a place where we train. It is where our life unfolds and develops. The dojang is a metaphor for the field of life itself. Everything that happens in our life will happen in the dojang. Any obstacle that we encounter in life we will encounter in the dojang, and we will see that it is not so much the obstacle that stops us, but our reaction to it. If we meet these obstacles head-on during training in the dojang, we will be ready when faced with them in our lives. That is why we must have the greatest humility and respect for our place of training, and each other."

Eventually, the day ended and soon I was driving home with my family. It had been a long day; everyone was tired and nodding off to sleep. I felt very peaceful and comfortable surrounded by them in the car, and I began to think about specific lessons I had learned during my years training as a martial artist in my dojang.

One of the first things I discovered about myself during my training was that I always wanted to do my best and be the best in everything I did. I had a very strong will to succeed and great perseverance in striving towards my goals. To accomplish one's goals, whether it be in the martial arts or any other field, it is essential that you know your limitations and strengths. Growth of self-awareness, particularly in the martial arts, is probably the most important aspect in the development of the life of a martial artist.

The martial arts itself is a system that very clearly understands strengths and weaknesses. The human body is a natural weapon and the martial arts teach how to use this natural weapon to its greatest advantage. During training, the student quickly becomes aware of his or her natural strengths and weaknesses. For example, imagine a small-boned martial artist competing against a 250-pound strong man. This would be an obvious mismatch. Or would it?

Think of the possible strengths and weaknesses of both fighters.

Obviously, the large man would have the power and muscle mass over the smaller; yet, the smaller man would have the advantage of speed and agility. Both have common weak spots in the eyes, ears, throat, temples, and solar plexus. An attack on any one of these parts by either fighter could render the other defenseless. Knowledge of one's strengths and weaknesses, and that of your opponent, could place the situation on equal ground. Therefore, it is important to know your natural strengths and work on perfecting them. There is a beautiful Zen story that illustrates this point.

One day, a Zen master was walking through the forest with his students when they spotted a pheasant on the trail walking awkwardly. On thin legs, the pheasant wobbled back and forth as if lugging a heavy, unbalanced weight. A student of the master began making fun of the pheasant, mocking it with his words and actions. The Zen master seeing this behavior in his student ran up to him waving a stick in his hand as if he were going to strike him in the legs saying, "Fly! Fly!" The student became flustered and said to the teacher, "What do you mean?" Then, the master ran towards the pheasant waving the stick. As the master approached the pheasant, it took a couple of short hops and then soared into the air away from the master. Returning to the students, he said, "You see, we all have our strengths and weaknesses. The pheasant can't walk very well, but can fly, and we can walk very well, but can't fly." The students nodded and understood the lesson.

During my years in training, I was never the strongest one in my dojang. I was muscular, but small, not so powerfully built like some others students. Yet, I did possess speed, and I learned that power comes through speed. Therefore, in my training, I did not emphasize working out with weights, attempting to build powerful muscles and increasing my size and muscle mass. Instead, I frequently ran wind sprints concentrating on improving my speed and reaction time. Also, I trained often on the parallel bars to increase the coordination between speed and agility. This type of training for myself proved effective, but for someone else, it might have been wrong. Extending this notion beyond the world of the dojang and my life as a martial artist, I realized that speed, agility, and quickness of thinking and action has also been a strong point in my life as well. I have always acted quickly when I am sure of the right action to take. I have learned that my strengths and weaknesses that I discovered on the mats are the same as in life. This self-knowledge has been invaluable to me.

At home that evening after the celebration, I felt very relaxed. The day was coming to a close. Yet, it was so memorable and had such a deep impact on me that I didn't want it to end. I wondered what could I do. I was given the opportunity to take stock of my life that day, and the conclusion that I came to was that I felt happy where I was. I had traveled a good road with all my heart. And thanks to those who helped me along the way, I had a great deal of success, happiness, peace in my life, and humility in my heart. That evening I slept very well.

The following day I returned to my school and my normal routine ready to begin another thirty years. The days began to effortlessly flow by.

However, one afternoon doing work in my office a few weeks later, a thought popped into my mind. Why not tour the world visiting the martial arts centers associated with my school? The thought surprised me and, at once, seemed crazy and inspired. I let the thought sit for a couple of days. Then, one evening I approached my wife.

Kwang was very supportive. We both thought it was a good idea, but with one minor alteration in the plan. Instead of being away for the entire year, I would travel two to three weeks a month every few months. I agreed. So, for the remainder of that year, I traveled around the world visiting martial arts centers. I traveled to the Caribbean, Canada, Europe, and Asia. At each center, the students and teachers helped celebrate my thirty years as an instructor in the martial arts. I spent time with the instructors at the schools and meeting and training new students. Everywhere I went the reception was wonderful. I had not been out like this for over ten years and enjoyed it tremendously.

While in Korea, I had an interesting experience. It just so happened that the 75th Lions Clubs International Convention was being held in Seoul when I was there. For some time, I had been involved with the Lions Club. In Seoul, I discovered that I was the only Korean living outside of Korea who had risen to become District Governor. I attended the convention and enjoyed the friendship of other Lions.

As all things come to pass, the year soon came to a close and once again I settled down at home in my school in New York City.

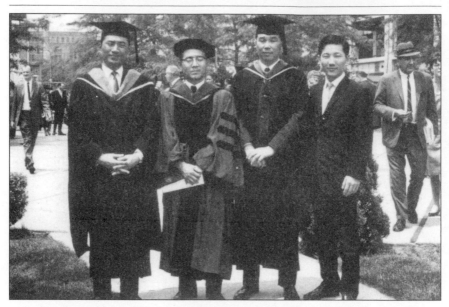

At his graduation from Long Island University. Richard Chun (left) and Professor of Economics Bum Sun Lee (second from left), 1965.

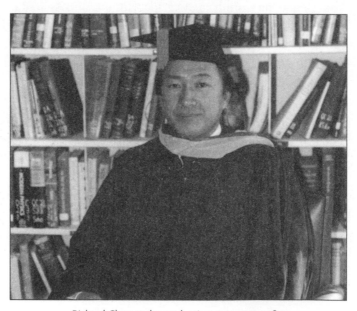

Richard Chun at the graduation ceremony, 1980.

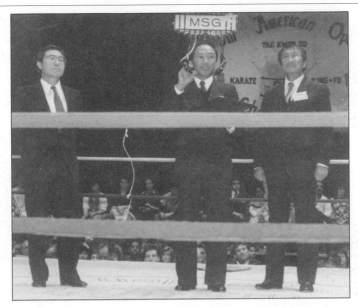

At the award presentation, Richard Chun (center), President of the United States Taekwondo Association, Special Assistant to the President of the World Taekwondo Federation; Grandmaster Ki Whang Kim (right); Grandmaster Henry Cho (left), Madison Square Garden, New York City, 1986.

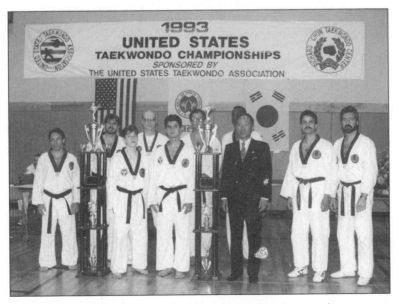

With the winners of the United States Taekwondo Championships.

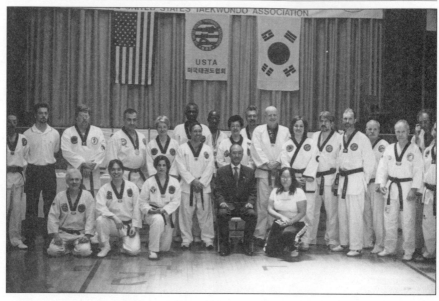

With master and senior instructors at the United States Taekwondo Championships, New York.

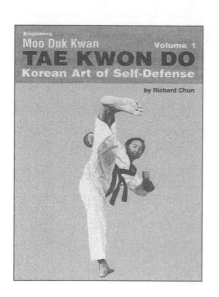

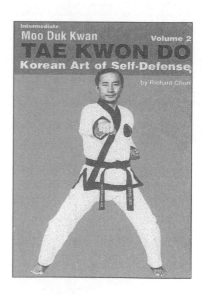

Covers of Richard Chun's third and fourth books on Moo Duk Kwan.

CHAPTER 11
A Lion and a Father

My father, Dr. Byung Hoon Chun, often gave free medical treatment to the financially needy in Seoul and on Cheju Island where he practiced medicine. Because of this generous service to others, he became well known among his patients and colleagues, quickly rising in his profession to become President of the Doctor's Association. The government of Korea also offered him a three-year appointment, along with 14 other top doctors in Korea, to serve as full colonel in the Army assigned to the Army Hospital in Seoul to recruit and train reputable, young doctors to serve in the military. Throughout his career as a doctor, he occasionally returned to the Army Hospitable to assist in the training of new doctors.

My father's generous service in the military and to the public certainly earned him wide respect. However, for the same reasons, he never became a very wealthy doctor. This never bothered him at all. All his life, he provided well for his family, a wife and eight children, and he was always an inspiring role model for his children in preparing us for a successful life. More than anyone I have ever known, my father had the biggest heart. All his life, he truly understood the meaning of giving, and this he passed on to his children.

Thus, when his best friend, also a colleague, approached my father with the idea of forming a Lions Club in Korea, he immediately jumped at the opportunity. Being the kind of man he was, the humanitarian ideals of the Lions Club greatly appealed to him. In the short few months that followed, he established the first Lions Club on Cheju Island and became its Charter President.

I was in Seoul at the time working at Air France, living with my brothers and sister when we heard about it. At that time, no one among us knew what the Lions Club was or did. In fact, we had never heard of it.

"It's an organization for service-minded people who want to work together," said my father. Then, he went on to explain how the club was the world's largest service organization, its motto and philosophy being 'we serve.'

"We will start by providing medical services for the needy by establishing free clinics," said my father.

"But you have been doing that already, Daddy," said my sister jokingly, and we all laughed.

"Yes, I know, but now it will be more organized," said my father, "and we will also be planting trees for the city streets and providing funds for park maintenance. We're even going to donate a large clock for the downtown area."

"It's great, Dad. We're proud of you," said my brother.

Back then, this was the extent of our knowledge and interest in the Lions Club. The fact that our father believed in it was sufficient enough for us. He remained a member and involved in the club's activities for the remainder of his life. My brother and sister took a sideline interest in it. For myself, it also remained solely on the periphery of my life. In fact, it was almost a decade later before I had my next contact with the Lions Club.

I had moved to New York by then, and my life was very active and busy, managing and teaching in my own martial arts school while attending university for an advanced degree. In my family, I was the second child to break away from the pack and live outside of Korea. First, my eldest brother moved to Tokyo to study and work. I went halfway around the world. This was a very big step; we were a close-knit family and remain so even to this day, but back then the physical distance seemed immense and communication between us naturally decreased, particularly during this developmental stage in my life. Even so, on a phone call with my father one day, he made the suggestion.

"Why not form a Lions Club in New York," he said. "It would be a way to meet new people."

"Oh, Dad, I'm really too busy these days," I said, "I don't know how I will find the time to participate, but for you, I'll look into it."

I truly didn't know where I would find the time, but these were not just idle words. Not long after the call, I contacted a local Lion's Club, mainly to appease my father and not really to benefit myself.

I looked up 'Lions Club' in a fund-raising brochure and made some inquiries. I informed them that I was a Korean martial artist living and teaching in the U.S. and that my father belonged to the Lions Club in Korea. They seemed genuinely interested, and before I knew it I had arranged to give demonstrations in a few clubs and at a district convention.

I remember the demonstration at the convention well. When I entered, I was greeted by a distinguished gentleman named Mr. Argento. He introduced himself as a District Governor in charge of seventy clubs. We conversed at a table where he pointed out the many plaques that had been awarded to him and the clubs under his jurisdiction. The plaques were from hospitals, city government offices, and youth organizations in appreciation for the services and funds that they had provided.

"Thanks to a fund raising drive last year, we were able to build a park in a low income area upstate," Mr. Argento said. "Now these children will have someplace to play ball."

He pulled out a photo album and pointed out some pictures showing a well-manicured baseball diamond and little leaguers in uniform with big grins on their faces.

"And tell me about your father's activities with the Lions Club in Korea," he asked.

I was stumped and embarrassed, because frankly, I didn't know any details about my father's activities with the Lions Club. I only knew that he belonged and was its charter president. Seeing the photos and talking to Mr. Argento suddenly put a human face on my father's activities during the past ten years.

I said something about donating a clock to the village square and he seemed impressed, not knowing that I was giving him information that was ten years old. In truth, I had no idea what my father did with the Lions Club, but began to understand the magnitude of his accomplishments. Suddenly I felt very proud of him, and wanted to know more about his activities, and about the Lions Club, in general.

"I know my father was very proud of being in a worldwide organization," I said. "Exactly how large is the Lions Club, Mr. Argento?"

"The Lions Club is now established in over 185 countries with one and a half million members," said Mr. Argento. "Lions are people who want to give something back to their communities and country by serving people in need. We enjoy working together to solve the major health and social concerns of our day, and we believe that by working in a group, our efforts and accomplishments can be magnified. We also enjoy the fellowship of being with others committed to service. People of all ages and backgrounds are Lions."

Our conversation ended and I gave the demonstration to the members. They all seemed to enjoy it and came up to me afterward to give me thanks.

After the demonstration, I thanked everyone and went home. I still was not sufficiently inspired to join the Lions Club at this time, but promised myself that I would look into it more seriously after my life and business were more established. I was inspired, however, to tell my father about my experience.

A few days later I wrote him and asked him about his activities with the Lions Club. I learned that the clinic he established ten years ago was still in operation, providing medical services to the people of Cheju Island. I learned that over the years his influence had spread well beyond his medical practice to include the entire city and community due to his involvement in the Lions Club. I learned that the clock that had been placed in the village square was still keeping time, although it had needed repairs from time to time. I wanted to know more and promised to keep in better touch.

"I will look into joining when my life settles down a bit, Dad," I replied. "I promise."

However, as usual for myself, the responsibilities of running a business soon took over again. I found it hard to keep in close contact, and before I knew it, I had slipped back to my normal routine, an occasional call here and there. A number of years went by before I heard news that changed things forever. The phone rang one evening. It was my brother. There hadn't been any communication between my family and myself for quite some time.

"Richard, how are you?" said my brother.

"I have been very busy; I hope you've been aware of that. Everything is going well, though. The school is progressing and I have been organizing a city-wide tournament, the first of its kind here," I said.

"Yes, we understand that you must be very busy. We are all proud of your accomplishments there."

We talked a little about the difference between life in America and Korea, and caught up on family news, what my brothers and sister was doing.

Then, suddenly, there was an uneasy silence on the phone.

"Kwang Moon, what's the matter?" I said.

"Richard, I'm calling to bring you bad news. I'm sorry to do it this way. We know that you must have so much on your mind."

"What's the matter?" I said again in a loud, impatience voice.

"Father passed away recently. It was sudden."

"What do you mean recently? When? I want to come home to see him before..."

"It was three months ago," my brother interrupted. "We decided not to tell you then because we knew you must have been in the middle of a school semester and with your martial arts school, you possibly could not afford the time to come home. We decided to wait until now. I'm so sorry."

I was stunned and speechless, and felt like I had been hit with a devastating blow. I felt rage well up inside of me and thought that I could never forgive my family for this.

"How could you do this to me?" I yelled into the phone.

As I said this, letting out all the anger, I understood that their actions were not out of disrespect for me, but out of genuine concern and love for my well being. With that thought, I felt my rage subside and an overwhelming sadness overcame me.

When the call ended, I felt very alone in my apartment, thousands of miles away from my family. I felt as small and vulnerable as a leaf in the wind, being blown about in a storm of emotions. I looked around my apartment for anything that represented my father, something that would connect me to him again. My mind seemed overwhelmed, blocked. Then, I saw it. The small painting that he sent to me, that I had framed, and was now hanging on the wall. It was a scenic landscape in the Chinese style of landscape paintings. My father's hobby was painting and calligraphy in this style. I gazed upon the painting as if I were looking at him. Then, I began to remember. All the memories of a father that come to you at a time like this poured into my mind, along with all that had been left unsaid and undone between us. Part of me—the stoic, disciplined warrior—responded to my loss with a detachment and understanding, yet soon all my defenses broke down like an old building crumbling in the raging waters of a flood. Through these cracks, the pain and sadness poured in, until finally I put my head in my hands and cried and cried for the longest time.

It took me about three months to forgive my family, and another decade before I had my next contact with the Lions Club. This time, however, it was for good.

I was 38 years old and the year was 1973. I had been in the U.S. almost 11 years. I was now married with a wife, daughter, and a newborn baby son. My martial arts school was now well established, and I had earned an advanced degree from the university. Life seemed finally secure and stable. In this more relaxed state of mind, certain feelings began to surface that could not in the turbulence of my earlier, growth years.

First, I began to feel that I wanted to give something back to the community. Second, I felt the need to assist other Koreans who were just starting out here in America. I didn't know in what form I would help. Then, one day, the thought and presence of my father came to me and I couldn't get him out of my mind. He seemed to be with me the whole day.

I saw his image again very clearly: a man of medium height, solid build and very handsome. He always well dressed and tidy in neat, clean pressed clothes. He was impeccably groomed, exuding the air of a military man and in some ways he always was: disciplined, strict, and conservative. Yet, what I remember most about him most was his kindness, his generosity, and his love for family and community life. He loved his work as a physician and worked hard at it, always sacrificing for others welfare. I also remembered his work with the Lions Club and the words he once asked me to consider.

"I believe the Lions Club is an organization that you would like," he said. "I think I know you by now, and feel that their goals and activities would fit with yours. Think about becoming a Lion."

I remembered that years before he passed away, I promised him that when my life was more settled, I would look into joining the Lions Club. Well, now I had no excuse. I decided that day to follow through on my promise to my father and myself.

First I spoke to a few Korean friends about the need in the New York Korean community to help newly-arrived immigrants get settled in such a large, unfamiliar city. We decided that we would form a group to help them. I brought up the idea of the Lions Club and explained a bit about it. They all seemed interested in hearing more, so we decided to invite someone from the Lions Club to talk to us about it. Over the next few days, I contacted several clubs and was able to locate someone who was authorized to promote the Lions Club by the International Association of Lions Clubs in Chicago.

A few days later, Mr. O'Rourke, a tall, well-built man in his fifties and District Governor of the New York City Chapter, met us at a neighborhood Korean restaurant in midtown Manhattan. He was accompanied by two club members. During dinner, Mr. O'Rourke and his associates spoke to us about the history, role, and ideals of the Lions Club.

"The Lions Club was established in 1917," said Mr. O'Rourke, "by a Chicago businessman named Melvin Jones, who believed that businessmen should not only be concerned with their business, but also with the betterment of their communities and society as a whole."

"A very worthy ideal," said one of my Korean friends.

"Absolutely," said one of Mr. O'Rourke's associates. "Since that time, the

Lions Club has grown steadily throughout the world with over 45,000 chapters presently established."

We all sat and listened with interest. Of course, our concern was to find a way to assist Koreans here in New York make a smoother transition from life in Korea to life in America.

"How do you decide in which ways you will serve your community or what projects you will work on?" I asked.

"Often through our own inspiration or what we perceive to be a need," said Mr. O'Rourke.

It was precisely the answer I wanted to hear. Mr. O'Rourke continued.

"Presently, the Lions Club International has been on a campaign, called Sight Conservation, to rid the world of preventable blindness through education and health care services."

We were impressed.

"Do you know how this project began?" asked Mr. O'Rourke. He didn't wait for a response.

"In 1925, Helen Keller addressed a Lions Club convention in Ohio. There, she challenged the Lions to be 'knights of the blind in the crusade against darkness.' She so inspired everyone there that for the past sixty years we have been recognized throughout the world for our work for the blind and visually impaired."

"In addition to this, the Lions Club has participated in other health-related areas such as diabetes awareness, environmental issues, and youth programs," said Mr. O'Rourke's colleague.

Needless to say, we were very impressed and asked whether we could work with Korean immigrants in the United States.

"In the Lions Club, we have an expression known as 'Lionism,' which is behavior and activity based on our code of ethics. In essence, it is action based on a high standard of personal and moral strength, and involves giving to others. So, Mr. Chun, to answer your question. Yes," said Mr. O'Rourke.

When he said this, I felt as if I were listening to a great martial arts master. The words could have been the same. Mr. O'Rourke and his associates continued to speak about specific projects that their club had worked on during the past year: organizing a medical conference to raise awareness of risk factors for heart disease; sponsoring a campaign for teens against drunk driving; holding a fund raising event to benefit a home for the elderly. I began to think about my father with great pride and love, and before the end of dinner, I decided that I wanted to establish a club of my own in New York.

I spent the next few months promoting the idea among my Korean friends and acquaintances. We needed 20 people to establish our own club. The response was overwhelming. By early 1974, we established the first New York Korean American Lions Club with a membership of 40 people. I became its Charter President. Our primary activity would be to assist Koreans here in New York City and the surrounding area. I was highly motivated to do this because I remembered the support that I received when I first came to America from my relatives, friends, and Dr. Kim. It would be rewarding for me to provide that support for others now.

We began our work immediately. We helped Koreans obtain immigration papers and licenses for work, provided accounting services for individuals and businesses during tax time, and offered a jobs bulletin board. Of the 40 members in our club, 6 were doctors. In honor of my father, we established a medical clinic for Koreans. In less than a year, our membership grew to 70 and we had assisted hundreds of people already. We were solidly on our way to becoming a vital force in the Korean community. I can't tell you how happy I felt to be involved in this, not only because of the real help we provided others, but the bond and connection it gave me to my father.

He had been right, of course. He did know me well. Through the Lions Club, I experienced a heightened and expanded sense of service; I had found another channel, besides martial arts, through which to express myself. This made me very happy and gave me a feeling of strength and invincibility, not at all unlike what I felt as a martial artist. Through my training in the martial arts, I had already developed a strong sense of service that manifested itself in a desire to assist, teach, and lead others on their path of life. My martial arts school had been a vehicle for that and now, through the Lions Club, I had found another vehicle. My influence spread into larger circles. For the first time, I saw how this work sustained my father and how it was now sustaining me. I also saw, perhaps for the first time in my life, that I was very much like my father.

My life as a Lion brought me many wonderful experiences and accomplishments. For 15 years I worked as an active club member organizing programs, fund raising, and imbibing the ideals and ethics of Lionism into my life. This work culminated in 1988 when I was elected District Governor of the New York-Bermuda District. As District Governor for 1 year, I helped raise over $100,000 that we donated to the Eye Surgery Department of

Montefiore Hospital, Einstein University, in the Bronx to provide medical service for those with eye disease.

During my tenure as District Governor, I arranged for 40 financially needy patients to have free glaucoma and cataract surgery and treatment. I also sponsored many drug awareness seminars in New York City to help young people keep free from drugs, alcohol, and smoking.

It was my good fortune that during this time my accomplishments as a Lion was covered by some newspapers in New York and Korea, and apparently read by some concerned, influential people. As a result, I was chosen to receive some awards: the President's Award from the Lions Club International, Chicago, and the Korean President's Medal at the Korean Consulate in New York. For the Korean President's Medal, I was asked to attend an afternoon ceremony at the Consulate.

It was one of the most memorable days in my life. Four Koreans—all businessmen like myself—received the honors at a black tie celebration. I arrived with my family at the embassy for cocktail hour where we met the other award recipients and distinguished guests. Over 100 people were in attendance. Then, we adjourned to a large hall where the Consul General of the embassy presented us each with the award. We were thanked for our contribution and had a wonderful day.

It was during this time as a Lion that I discovered my talent for fund raising, and in 1992 I was appointed as one of 9 members to the International Fundraising Committee. It was a very special appointment because this committee was generally composed of past International Presidents. I was the only District Governor to be selected.

Our 3-year mission was to raise funds for Campaign Sight First, the program against preventable blindness. We had learned, and had all been moved, by the statistic that 80% of the blindness in the world is preventable, while only 20% is due to natural causes and accidents. In the 3 years of our tenure, we raised over $130 million worldwide and gave donations to 70 hospitals and government agencies.

Presently, my work with the Lions Club is more subdued, carrying on my responsibilities as Past District Governor. What I have learned over the years as a Lion is that the life of a Lion is based on love, sacrifice, and giving. To summon these qualities in my life in my role as a Lion was not at all difficult because I had already developed them in my life as a martial artist.

When a martial artist talks about his training and his goals, the first words that come to mind are patience, self-control, and humility. Yet, underlying these virtues, a truly developed martial artist must have a deep and enduring love for the practice and training, and the ability to sacrifice for it. It is a choice one makes, and it calls for hard work and disciplined action.

To tell yourself that you will commit at least 2 to 3 hours a day in training means that you must sacrifice other activities. It may mean not hanging out with friends at the mall one afternoon or seeing a film in the evening. This is not to say that there is no room in a martial artist's life for fun and enjoyment, just not at the expense of the desired goal. Remember, the path of a martial artist is not always easy, and it is not for everyone. But it is always rewarding, and the ultimate goal will be profound in its effect on your life.

This is the choice I made for myself. I followed that path with a full heart, and I am happy for it. However, the martial arts have not completely absorbed my life. There are many activities and hobbies that I have enjoyed throughout my life. I have found, however, that what I have learned as a martial arts master has always carried over to that new activity.

For example, I have always been an enthusiast of Badook (Go) in which I have progressed to 1st Kup. The levels in Chinese Chess are somewhat like the different colored belts of the martial arts. You start at the 10th Kup and work your way down over the years to the 1st. I used to play quite regularly with friends in Korea where my father, who was at professional level, taught me. Once I moved to the U.S., my playing subsided because not many people know the game, but occasionally I would find someone who knew how to play or on return trips to Korea.

Also, I play golf whenever I can. Being on the golf course is beautiful because it is an outdoor sport, unlike martial arts for the most part, and it is very expansive, using large open spaces. The concentration, patience, accuracy, and persistence that are necessary to play a good game of golf are qualities that are identical to those used and developed in the martial arts. I believe that these qualities have greatly enhanced my golf game.

In addition, I am a lover of opera and chamber music, and an avid ballroom dancer.

I have also been a devoted Christian for a long time, currently being a member of the Arcola Korean United Methodist Church in Arcola, New Jersey. Over the years, I have been involved with sending out missionary material to Asian, African, and Latin American countries.

So you see, a martial artist can lead a well-balanced life with numerous interests and activities. What you will find, I am sure, is that your practice of the martial arts will benefit everything you do. This is what I have always found.

Now, there is another part of my story that I have not talked much about, and at this point in my book, I think it is the right time to speak of possibly the greatest channel of expression in my life. That is my role as a family man: husband to my wife, father to my children, and part of a large extended family.

I have 5 brothers and 2 sisters. As our lives developed, I am proud to say that we all turned out fine, finding our paths in life and becoming successful people. One sister moved to the U.S. years after I arrived. She studied at Long Island University earning a Master's Degree in Library Science and worked for many years as a librarian. She now lives in Westchester, N.Y. with her family.

My mother actually passed away when I was five years old and my sister was three. We were too young to remember the event. I know her face only from photographs that my aunt showed me. My father remarried not too long after my mother's death. My brothers and other sister are, in reality, half brothers and sisters, but I never thought of them that way. We are all one strong, close family.

My eldest brother is a doctor who engaged in business for many years in Tokyo, and another brother is a Professor of Psychology at Yonsei University, my alma mater. In the line of our family, I came next. You know my story. A younger brother moved to California and runs a newspaper and another younger brother, who followed most closely in the footsteps of my father, became a dentist and practices on Cheju Island. My younger sister is married and lives in Seoul and, sadly, another brother passed away several years ago.

My stepmother also passed away a few years ago on Cheju Island, where she spent most of her days after we moved there during the war. Even though my brothers and sisters are spread out all over the world, I have always remained close to them.

My cousin in Washington, D.C., whom I stayed with briefly when I first arrived in America, was directly responsible for my meeting my wife. My cousin was a music professor at a women's college in Seoul, Ewha University, before she immigrated to the U.S. She remained close friends with the President of the college all her life. Years after I moved here, when I was ready to settle down, she arranged for me to travel to Korea to be introduced to some women I might be interested in. Unlike courting procedures in the U.S., this style of semi-arranged marriage was quite common in Korea. It is not as strict and formal as India where the parents do the choosing, but in Korea two people would be introduced for the very clear purpose of choosing a mate. The final choice would be up to the two individuals. I traveled to Seoul and visited Ewha University where I was introduced to numerous women.

I first met Kwang at the office of the Chairman of the Board. I remember she was a beautiful woman, somewhat shy, and very intelligent. She was an assistant to the Chief Administrator in charge of professors and students. I liked her right away, but at that time, she was meeting a doctor who studied in the United States. This, of course, made her unsure about me and I was also unsure of the situation.

Over the next few weeks, I met about 20 other ladies who were all good women and would be excellent mates, but there wasn't one that stood out. It seemed to me that I would be going back to the U.S. without having met the right woman. I was planning to head home in about a week. Interestingly, a friend suggested I meet one other lady.

That afternoon, I dressed in a fine suit and went to the Chosen Hotel, a luxurious hotel in downtown Seoul, to meet this final lady. I was waiting anxiously when Kwang approached. I was taken aback to see her. We both where aware that we were set up for a second date. I was even more surprised to see that she had brought her parents and sister to meet me.

"I guess it's fate that we meet again," I said, with a smile on my face.

She introduced me to her parents and sister, and we sat and talked for a while until her father suggested that she and I spend some time alone together. We decided that we would take a walk around Namhan Sansung, a castle on the top of a mountain that overlooked the city of Seoul. It was a beautiful spot and very romantic, particularly on an early summer day when all the trees were in blossom. The air was filled with sunlight, warmth, and birdsong. There, we walked and talked for a while.

"What about the doctor you are dating from the United States?" I asked her at one point.

Our conversation and walk was sweet. We decided that we would see each other again soon. A few days later, we saw a show together at the Walker Hill resort. I remember being absorbed in the show and Kwang had noticed my focused attention and concentration. These qualities impressed her. On the following day we went again to the castle where I proposed marriage. We announced it to our families, and I postponed my return flight home. In three weeks our families and friends joined us at the beautiful and elegant restaurant in the Korean Airline Building, which we rented for our engagement party. We were married eight months later at a ceremony with friends and family back in the United States.

This may sound like a whirlwind romance and this type of courtship may seem foreign to westerners, yet I am happy to say that I have been married to Kwang now for 30 years. She's not only a wonderful wife, but my best friend, confidant, and also my business associate. Without her in my life as my wife and friend, I could have never become the man I am. And, without her help running my business as she has done over the years, I could have never been as successful.

Together, we have two children: my son Yong Taik or 'Ray' as we call him is a graduate of M.I.T. with a Master's Degree in Electrical Engineering. Currently, he is working for his own company. My daughter Kyung Mee or 'Kay', is a graduate of Wellesley College and the French Culinary School. She is working for *"Real Simple Magazine"* as the Senior Associate Food Editor.

My relationship with my son and daughter has been like that of a friend as well as a parent. Communication with them has been easy and we even joke with each other frequently like good friends. My children have also taken an interest in my life. They are both trained in the martial arts and have progressed to black belt status. They still come to the school for special events and to help us occasionally with the business.

I can't tell you how proud I am of my children and how much I love my family. These feelings go deeper than I can ever imagine, and I am forever grateful to them for that. My family has always supported me completely in my love and work as a martial artist and a Lion. We have shared so much together, and I'm sure their presence in my life has helped shape me into who I am. I only hope that my family will be as proud of me as I am of my father.

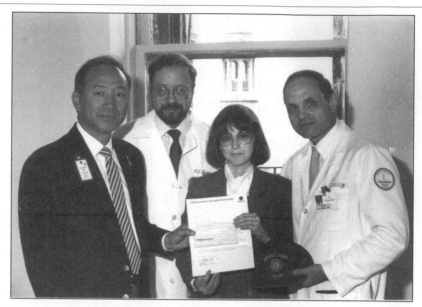

Richard Chun, District Governor of New York—Lions Clubs International, donating a big check to establish and advanced eye surgical laboratory at Montefiore Hospital in Bronx, N.Y., 1988.

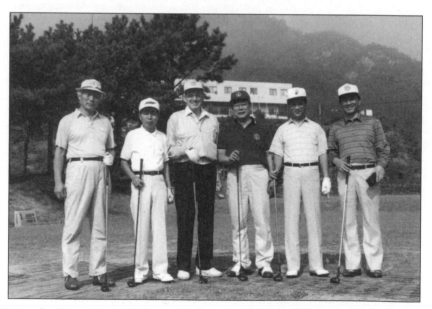

During the Olympic Games in Korea, 1988. From the left, Richard Chun; Lion director and congressman Il Yoon Kim; Director Dr. Yo Chull Shin; President of the Lions Clubs International Association Austin Jennings; Director Min Koo Kang; C.C. Kim-D.G., at Yusong Country Club, Daejon, Korea.

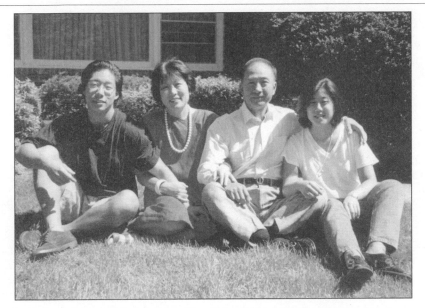

Chun's family from the left; Ray, Kwang Hae, Richard Chun, and Kay at home in New Jersey.

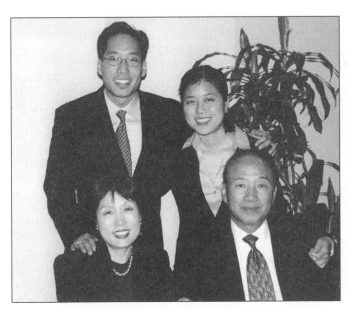

Chun's family from the left above; Ray, Kay, Kwang Hae, and Richard Chun at
USTA headquarters in New York.

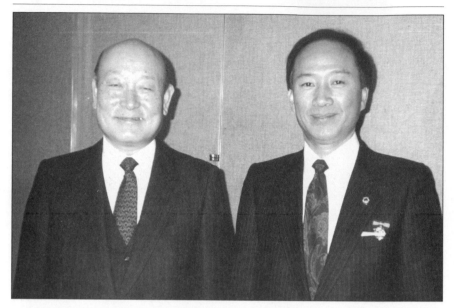

At the award ceremony, Honorable Ambassador Ro Myung Kong (left), and Richard Chun, receiving the Presidential Special Award for Outstanding Humanitarian Services, New York City, January, 1989.

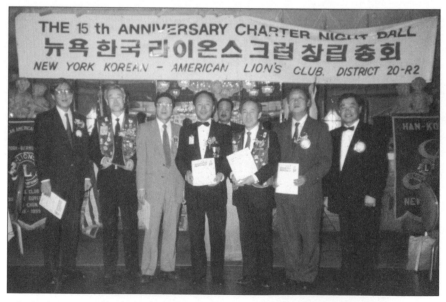

At the Anniversary Charter Night Ball for the New York Korean-American Lions Club for which Richard Chun (center) served as the Charter President.

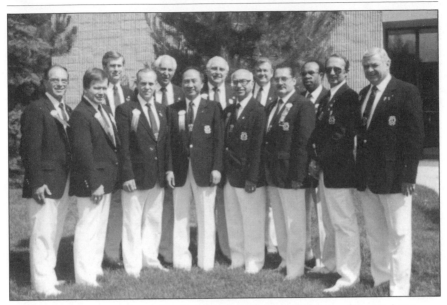

Richard Chun (fourth from left) with the Council of District Governors of New York State, 1988-1989.

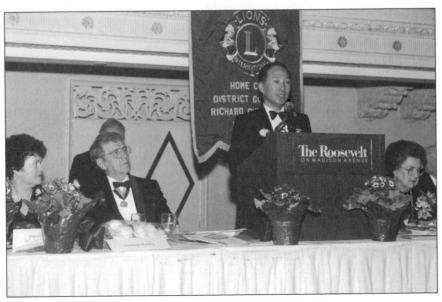

Addressing the New York District Convention, District Governor Richard Chun (center), International President of the Lions Clubs International Association Austin Jennings (left), past International President Robert J. Uplinger (right), 1988.

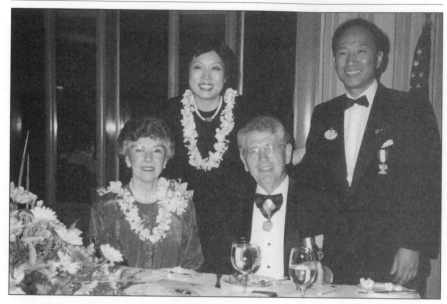

With International President of the Lions Clubs International Association Austin Jennings and Carmine, District Governor Richard Chun and Kwang Hae, 1988.

CHAPTER 12

The Way of the Warrior

There is a famous 16th Century Chinese painting by T'ang Yin titled "Dreaming of Immortality in a Thatched Cottage." The painting depicts a monk sitting by an open window in a cottage atop a mountain. His hands are covering his face and he is lost in contemplation. Off to the left, we see the same monk flying in a standing position over a vast expanse of mountain ranges, his long hair and robe trailing behind him in the wind like out-stretched wings. The painting has a great feeling of openness, freedom, and joy.

The painting also expresses something fundamental in the life of a martial artist. That is the desire to achieve something beyond our pre-conceived ideas and notions. It is impossible to fly. Yet, the monk sees himself soaring effortlessly over the mountaintops. Likewise, the martial artist sees himself achieving heights of physical excellence and prowess as to render himself completely invincible to his opponents, so invincible in body and mind that he is immortal.

The reality is that in both situations—that of the monk and the martial artist—they truly believe their goal is attainable. The monk strives towards his goal through meditation and contemplation; the martial artist through hard work and discipline, always pushing himself to his limits. A maxim from the martial art tradition says that 'tomorrow's battle is won in today's training.' How true this is, and even at a young age, I understood the value of hard work and the idea of pushing beyond one's limits.

Occasionally after practice at the Moo Duk Kwan Institute, a few of my fellow students and I would stay on for some "overtraining," as we called it.

"Now be careful, boys," said Master Hong as he left the gym. "Know when to push yourself and also when to stop."

Master Hong was aware of our occasional overtraining, and he approved of it. Although not actually part of our official training, he knew that over-training was necessary and even encouraged us. So, on our own every few months or so, we stayed on after practice or met on a Saturday or Sunday morning to workout strenuously. We knew on these days that we were going to test ourselves beyond our capabilities. So, we had to be ready, physically and psychologically. We devised a variety of ways to overtrain. Sometimes, we would go into the mountains outside of Seoul and run barefoot along a path to develop and control balance and grace in our movements. At times, we focused on sheer speed, racing along mountain paths, hopping branches, dodging stones, and weaving around trees and bushes. Other times, we concentrated just on kicking our knees as high as we could while running through the forest. We might conclude the workout with bouts of stick fighting or attempting to break the thin slate stone that we found along the river banks. One of us would hold one end of the stone up while the other end rested on the ground. We would increase the thickness of the stone until it became impossible to break. Many times, however, we just stayed in the gym after all the students had left.

"... and please remember to lock the door, " Master Hong would always say, just before leaving.

By ourselves in the empty gym, we might attempt breaking techniques on boards or kicking as high as we could in the air. Many times, we would spar—all out—for 40 minutes, which was 10 minutes more than our normal 30. In order to push ourselves even more, one of us would be chosen to spar for the full amount of time while the others played a sort of tag team, therefore always remaining fresh. After those 40 minutes, you had seen everything and were close to exhaustion. In six months, you would do it again to see what progress you had made.

Why did we do this?

The answer is simple: just to do more. It is natural to want to do more, to test yourself and your capabilities. This is how you progress.

Even to this day in my school, I practice this philosophy. The only difference being that now, it is me who is saying "be careful, be careful" as I encourage my students to push themselves to their limits. Often, during warm-ups or calisthenics, I will push a student to do 110 sit-ups when I know their limit is 100 or to break 7 boards when their limit is 6.

Overtraining creates something unique in the psychology. First, there is the on-the-spot pressure to achieve. Sometimes, we respond better under pressure, digging down deeper into ourselves to elevate our performance. Second, and equally important, occasional overtraining teaches us to maintain a strong work habit, to fulfill our duty and responsibility to ourselves to work hard, so that when we are called upon to perform a task under pressure, we do respond. And third, of great value, overtraining is really a tool for teaching us to always be positive because there will be times when we push ourselves to our limits, and we fail. We must learn that failure is part of the process and that we should always keep a positive attitude so that next time the situation arises, we will succeed.

Often during the course of training for a young martial artist, fear and lack of confidence arise. One might face their fears when asked to perform that which seems out of their range of capabilities.

It is important never to let fear conquer us, whether it is in training or in life. Fear and negativity can easily defeat us, and many times, is the culprit in slowing down our progress, not to mention destroying life-long dreams. Fear disrupts our inner state of balance and integrity, and only fosters inaction. You must find a way to overcome your fears. I believe training in the martial arts is a classroom lesson in overcoming fears.

I can't tell you how many times I felt fear pounding in my heart when I had to perform a daunting task or face a formidable opponent. Also, I can't tell you how many times a student of mine expressed their fears to me for these same situations. We have all been through it; it is part of life. Yet, there are definite ways to defeat fears, rather than let fear defeat you:

Rule number 1: Realize that in many cases, fear is an illusion created by you. This is particularly true when it comes to our experiences in training. Remember that training is just that—training. It is the time and place when we explore, experiment, take chances. There is room in training for a lifetime of successes and failures. No one, certainly not even the greatest warriors, has gone through life without their share of wins and losses.

In the great scripture of Yoga and enlightenment of ancient India, the *Bhagavad-Gita*, there is a verse that states:

Perform actions having abandoned attachment
and having become balanced in success and failure.

Once we accept the fact that on the mat, we will win and lose many times. What is our concern is to work hard and try to do our best every time we perform. When we do this, we will find that we begin to win more times than lose. And more importantly, we grow in our art. In this state, fear ceases to exist.

This verse also brings out another subtle point in its reference to 'abandoning attachment.' This simply means that we do not engage in action solely for the end result. Certainly, it is right to work towards a goal, but you must enjoy the process, or else you will find yourself becoming bored, angry or frustrated. When your attention is on the process, you will accomplish two goals: first and foremost, the enjoyment of the activity and second, the rewards or fruits of your work.

Rule number 2: Fear is defeated by knowledge and experience. A sure-fire method to face your fears head on is to clearly identify your fear and then set out to understand it. Once you begin to understand the fear, you will quickly see that it was baseless or that you have gained enough information to face it.

This method proved true for me many times. It often came up in competition and tournaments when I felt the pressure and fear to win. Particularly because I hated to lose. My approach would be to learn as much about my opponents as I could before stepping out on the mat with them. Once I observed and became aware of their strengths and weaknesses, I knew what to expect and what my strategy would be. It always put me on solid ground. Knowledge has a way of bringing your fears down to earth where you have a much better chance of battling them.

Experience goes hand in hand with knowledge. In some respects, they are the two sides of the same coin. With time, as you experience the same things over and over, your knowledge of the situation automatically grows and fear spontaneously dissipates.

I'm sure we all have had the experience of meeting a neighbor's big dog for the first time. The dog rushes up to you, barking loudly and fiercely. You stand rigid with all your senses on red alert. But then, once the dog gets to know you and becomes familiar with you over time, you and the dog become good buddies. Soon, it is hard to even imagine that first fearful interaction with him.

Rule number 3: Fear melts away with preparation. For about twenty years now, I have been a professor of physical education at Hunter College, City University of New York. Besides teaching martial arts, I lectured on all aspects of physical training and fitness as well as sports psychology. When I first began my career as a professor, I was apprehensive about my ability to speak in front of people. I was experienced in teaching martial arts, but that had always involved teaching something concrete and physical on the gym floor in my toboks. I felt confident about myself in this arena. However, teaching concepts behind a podium in front of a class full of students was a different thing. I didn't know how my students would respond, especially being that English was my second language. These considerations, of course, were not going to deter me. I decided that mastery of my material and preparation for my classes would be essential.

I worked hard for every class, mastering the material as fully as I could, thinking out the proper approach to present it, and trying to anticipate every question that would be raised. Of course, there were surprises and, at times, I was forced to be spontaneous and think on my feet, but I can definitely say that proper preparation helped me overcome any fear I had to teach and speak in front of people. Now, it comes comfortably and easy to me.

I learned that the more you know your subject and the more you feel comfortable with yourself, you will be able to present information to others in a lively and informative way. In general, whenever you feel fearful about an impending event or task ahead of you, do everything you can to prepare for it. Preparation will give you the necessary ammunition and self-confidence to overcome any fears. It worked well for me.

I often taught these rules and other aspects of the mental training to my students during question and answer periods we would have in class.

Many times, my students would ask very provocative and probing questions that brought out beautiful points about being a martial artist. One question in particular stands out in my mind that a recently promoted black belt student asked one day.

"Master Chun," he said, "if there were four people together and one of them was a master of the martial arts, would you be able to tell who the master was?"

"Oh yes," I joked, "the one wearing the black belt."

The students laughed.

"But seriously now, that is a very interesting question. And, I think the answer is yes. If the four are presented naturally—that is we are not seeing them in a fighting situation—I would say that the master in the martial arts would be the one who is the most humble, the most modest."

"Why is that?" another student asked.

"Because the master doesn't need to show off. They are self-possessed; he or she knows what they can do. It is not in their nature to show off, physically or verbally. The true martial artist always waits and sees if action if necessary; if it is, then their action is precise and deliberate. The master of the martial arts will always be the one who radiates a quiet calm and dignity."

It was a beautiful question and I remembered feeling inspired by it. I continued, teaching them about the essence of what is called warrior elegance.

A master of the martial arts cultures a certain elegance in their life. This elegance is based upon their inner strength, sense of duty and responsibility, and strong moral character. Outwardly, it is expressed through their physical grace and posture. Remember, they are well-trained and in excellent shape. In some ways they are like dancers, masters of movement. They exude or radiate refinement and dignity. This has become their being, who they are. This is what the master of the martial arts gives to the world—the true meaning of self-esteem and dignity. You can feel that in their presence.

"We see that in you, Master Chun," a student remarked.

"Yes, yes," other students added.

Feeling proud and slightly embarrassed, I thanked my students for their compliments and bowed to them in respect.

Speaking to my students about warrior elegance set my mind thinking. Questions that I have thought about ever since.

Do I possess this elegance that I talk about? Do I radiate self-confidence and dignity to those around me? Have I truly accomplished the goals of a martial artist in my lifetime? What more is there for me to accomplish?

These questions are not easily answered, particularly when directed at yourself, and certainly not answered in one day. These are questions to be pondered over time.

I have spent my life in the pursuit of the martial arts. I am a ninth degree Grandmaster in Taekwondo with mastery in hundreds of forms. I have taught for over forty years, passing my knowledge on to hundreds, maybe thousands, of students. From a purely technical point of view, I still engage in practice and research of the forms. I am still learning new forms and I am constantly refining and creating new ones and experimenting with sequencing of forms. I hope through my work in this area to push the art of Taekwondo, in some small way, to its limits, therefore playing a role in its evolution as a martial art.

Yet, it is the area of moral development that I am most concerned with. Here, of course, there is always room for growth. Being the best possible human being that I can be is the most important thing in my life as a man and as a martial artist. I try to always set a good example to others in my life. I strive to be a good person, good teacher, good husband, good father. I do my best to serve and give something to my community. Above all, I desire balance and integration in my life. This is my essence. This is what I attempt to be and to teach.

The timeless symbol of yin/yang expresses this philosophy. The perfect circle expressing wholeness—the wholeness of man, of woman, of family, of country, of humanity, of nature, of the cosmos. Yet, this wholeness is divided into parts, two equal parts, perfectly complimenting each other.

The central concept expressed in the yin/yang symbol is the concept of balance. Even visually, from whatever perspective you view the symbol, it is balanced to the eye. Yet, what does this balance represent? What is being balanced within it? The answer is simple and vast. Everything. Every living and non-living entity, every concept and notion, whatever exists in idea and form falls within its range. The yin/yang symbol swallows up extreme to extreme—white/black,

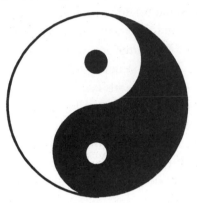

Yin and Yang Symbol

man/woman, earth/sky, laughing/crying, love/hate, giving/taking, everything/nothing. But, how does this relate back to us, our experience? For me, it means many things, affecting both the mind and behavior. For example, if someone hates you, try to love them. If you get something from someone, give something back. If you are active, get some rest. Yin/yang is a fundamental principle in life and is everywhere.

I first learned of yin/yang during my training in the martial arts. I learned that where there is offense, there is also defense. I learned to kick and simultaneously use my arms and body to maintain balance. I learned to inhale and exhale breath appropriately. I learned to develop a strong body and a strong mind. I learned that there are obstacles and the action to overcome obstacles. I learned to defeat fear with confidence.

For the youth who are starting on the path of a martial artist, I want to emphasize to you that it will take a long time to achieve your goal, to become a master. There is no shortcut on this path, and this is true in other fields of endeavor as well. A goal worth striving for is a goal well worth the hard work and time spent. In the process, something unique and special will happen to you. You will develop good habits in life and learn to overcome bad ones. Imagine being so preoccupied with the positive things in your life that you do not even have the time for anything negative. This will happen. Also, you will develop discipline and balance in life, outer and inner, physically and morally. You will have a strong self-identity and earn the respect of others, while spontaneously growing in leadership abilities. Most importantly, you will possess self-knowledge, which is the secret of self-control and mastery in life. As a master of the martial arts, know that you always carry with you a powerful tool—yourself—that you constantly use to better yourself.

The martial arts, however, is not just for the youth. All ages can benefit.

For the middle-aged and the elderly who are considering taking classes in the martial arts or just beginning your practice, you will quickly find an improved state of health and growth in self-confidence. For many people, growing older is often accompanied with failing health, loneliness, and fears; it generally brings more rigidity in body and mind. Instead of entering into this time of life with wisdom, strength and security, they find themselves frail and fearful. Add to this condition the underlying fear of death, and the situation quickly becomes depressing. A time of life which should be spent in peace and comfort is instead spent in despair. This does not have to be the situation.

Practice in the martial arts is the perfect antidote to this condition of the elderly. First of all, don't think that you are too old to begin training in the martial arts. I have had numerous students over the years who started at a late age, and they progressed well using their experience and maturity to their advantage. The training needn't be too strenuous and is often geared towards age considerations. I always emphasize to my elderly students never to strain and to take their workouts at a comfortable pace. Don't postpone it because you feel you are too old. It doesn't matter when you start; you will soon notice results. You will find yourself becoming more outgoing, more spontaneous, healthier, and less fearful.

At this point in my story, close to its end, I feel that I must talk briefly about the connection between the martial arts and the fear of death, philosophy and religion.

I do realize that the experience of growing older and dealing with issues of aging, including facing one's own mortality, is intimately tied to religious beliefs and points of view. I firmly believe that these beliefs, in conjunction with the physical and mental well-being that the martial arts brings, are very powerful tools to bring into our later years for our health and happiness.

Recently, I had a experience that verified this.

In the fall of 1997, I went through a series of medical tests for problems I was having with my lungs. It seemed that every fall and winter for the past few years, I couldn't resist coming down with the flu accompanied by a deep, nagging cough, despite getting a flu shot. During the months when my doctor was performing tests to determine a diagnosis, I went through a very stressful time. The possibilities for my diagnosis ranged from a previous case of pneumonia that may have caused permanent damage to my respiratory system to the more life-threatening diagnosis of lung cancer. These possibilities scared me and I spent many nights awake and worried. Did I sustain permanent damage that would affect my ability to teach and train? Did I have cancer and would I have to go through the debilitating treatment of chemotherapy? Was I ready to face my own mortality? It was a time of deep soul-searching.

Being a martial artist, I knew that I had spent my entire life in a practice that created a healthy body and mind. There was no reason my body should break down now. I felt connected to that intelligence in my body and mind that maintains one's health, and I wouldn't allow negative thoughts to overthrow me. Instead, I held onto a belief in my innate ability to heal and be healthy, to overcome any obstacle, including my own health problems.

In addition to my belief in my physical well-being, I am a religious man. I prayed on my own and I also enlisted the prayers of my family and members of my church. These prayers brought much comfort to me during this time. Knowing that so many others were putting their attention on my situation was a very powerful experience. I could almost feel the change inside me from their prayers. Tapping deeply into my religious nature at this time also helped me to surrender to God's will. I grew in the belief that the best and right thing would happen to me through mine and others prayers.

The powerful tradition of the martial arts also helped me through this time. In the philosophical tradition of Taekwondo, there is a belief that an underlying oneness in nature exists at the center of all life, a oneness that gives rise to a benevolent force which guides and directs all our actions and is the source of our strength and wisdom. To the degree that you are connected with this force is the degree to which you are invincible and immortal. It is the healing and life-giving fountain within us. In essence, a master of the martial arts is one who has knowledge and experience of this oneness. To realize it is the ultimate goal of a martial artist. I don't know if this concept is where my religious beliefs as a Christian merge, but I do know that I believe in it, its power, and have sensed its truth in my life. It is what I am and what I have become, whether I call myself a religious warrior or a GrandMaster Christian. It doesn't matter either way. I'm grateful for these two powerful streams in my life. I'm sure that they helped me during this time.

After more than three months of physical testing and psychological stress, my doctors finally arrived at a diagnosis. There was a bacteria in my lungs that had caused the problem; it was not serious, and would be treated with an antibiotic. So that was it, a simple condition with an easy conclusion. Needless to say, I felt great relief. I also knew that my belief in myself as a master in the martial artist and as a religious man either saved me or pulled me through these trying times.

The experience also set me thinking. A day will come when it is my time to say good-bye, permanently, to the beauty and miracle of what we call life. I am not immortal. We are not immortal. Like the monk in the painting, we only see ourselves flying over the mountain ranges; it is in our imaginations only. But, it does not mean that we failed. On the contrary, my immortality is real in the memories of those I have touched in my lifetime and in the legacy of the tradition of which I have been a part. I only hope that when that final day comes, I will feel the inner strength to face it clearly and with dignity. I believe that all I have done in life and become in life has been a part of that whole, that oneness, for the good of myself and all. This is the only true preparation, I think.

Last year, my great teacher, Master Hong, passed away. I was not able to return to Korea to pay my respects, yet I felt the loss deeply and took time to privately mourn. Even though he is gone from us, his presence lives on and he continues to give me the right direction as a human being and a warrior.

I am fortunate in the life that I have lived. I am healthy and happy. I have given of myself, 100 percent of the time, to my path and life as a martial artist and man. Everyday has brought me some happiness and growth, and as a result, I feel that I have become, to the highest degree that I could, a master of my own life and destiny.

I thank God for this gift. I thank my martial art Masters for this gift. I thank my family and all my friends. I thank my students, and I thank myself.

This has been my life, a life of a martial artist.

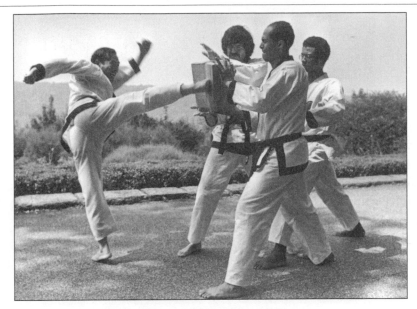

Richard Chun with his black belt students, 1968.

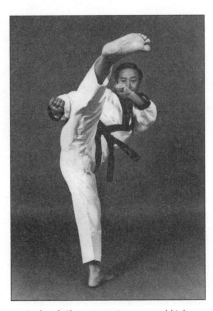

Richard Chun executing a round kick.

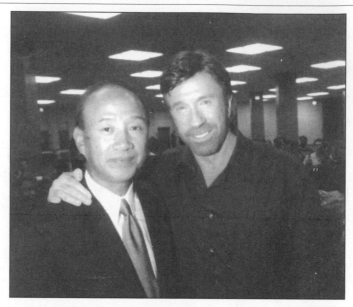

With actor and master Chuck Norris, Madison Square Garden, New York City, 2000.

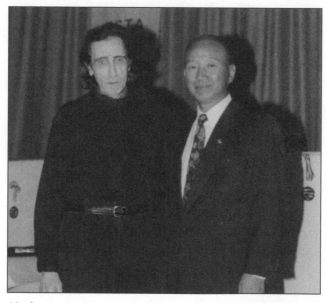

With the world's famous martial arts promoter Aaron Banks at the USTA Championships, New York, 2002.

Postscript

At the conclusion of my writing this book, I was fortunate to have one of the most memorable and joyful experiences in my life. As if the full and perfect blossoming of a flower took place at just the right time, and as if this blossoming was the perfect reward for my years of work putting my life down into words, I took a very special trip back to Korea.

This trip was different from the others that I had taken over the years because on this journey, I was accompanied by 30 of my students. Both men and women of different levels of martial art accomplishment, ranging in ages from 15 to 65—these were students from New York and New Jersey that I had trained and watched grow over the years.

The purpose of our trip was two-fold: First, to further our training of advanced techniques in sparring, forms, self-defense and meditation from well-known masters. We were preparing for the 2000 U. S. Taekwondo Championships, sponsored by the United States Taekwondo Association, to be held in May in New York City. The second reason for our trip was so my students could immerse themselves in the people and culture of Korea, the homeland of our sport and art.

For 10 days we trained at a famous university in Seoul which specializes in physical education and specifically offers Taekwondo as a major in their curriculum. Our instructors were the great masters of the day and our classmates were the Korean National team, which included many Olympians who competed in 1996. I knew many of the Olympians and masters there because for about 25 years, I served the World Taekwondo Federation as an international referee and was recently promoted to WTF-H Class in January, 2000. Four to six hours a day we trained with these learned teachers and students in the advanced techniques of kicking and sparring.

We did find time in our schedule to enjoy shopping at the famous Itaewon and visit the Duk Soo Palace in Seoul where the emperors of the great Korean dynasties ruled for many centuries. One day, we took a four hour bus trip to Kyung Ju, a historical city where the founder of Taekwondo, Hwarang-Do, trained. There, in the silent, peaceful atmosphere of the Bulkuksa Temple, we meditated.

We also spent some hours with Dr. Kim, who spoke eloquently about the history and growth of Taekwondo. His words never failed to motivate. Each student received from Dr. Kim a set of cuff links and a watch to remind us of our time in Korea.

During these 10 days, I felt as if I had entered Heaven. I was overcome by gratitude and respect, and silenced by the joy of being with my students in my homeland. On one side were my students and all they were learning and experiencing. On the other side were the great masters and practitioners of Taekwondo in Korea today. I was like a conduit between them, a conductor of the life and principles of this tradition coming from Korea itself, through me to my students.

I only hope that this book accomplished the same for you.

Last May, I celebrated my 40th anniversary as instructor / owner in my own school. We held the 2002 Annual United States Invitational Taekwondo Championships in New York City. The world famous martial arts promoter, Aaron Banks, presided over the event. I saw many of my black belt students, who started with me when they were young, and who have now gone on to open their own schools. I noticed their graying hair and mature look and marveled at the passing of time.

After 40 years of teaching in the United States, after 55 years of practicing martial arts, after 67 years of life, I still love what I am doing and feel that I am still growing strong.

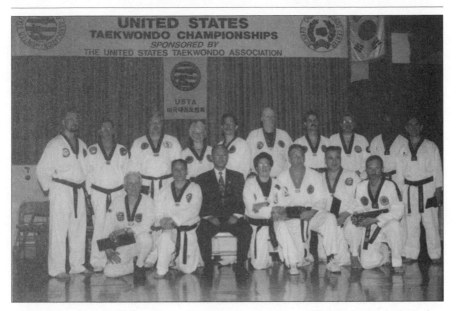

With master and senior instructors at the USTA championships, celebrating Richard Chun's fortieth anniversary teaching Taekwondo in America, 2002.

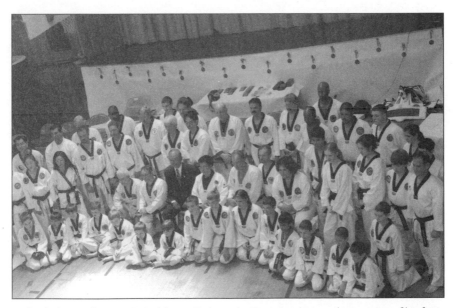

Richard Chun at the 2002 United States Taekwondo Championships on the occasion of his fortieth anniversary teaching Taekwondo in America, New York City, May 5, 2002.

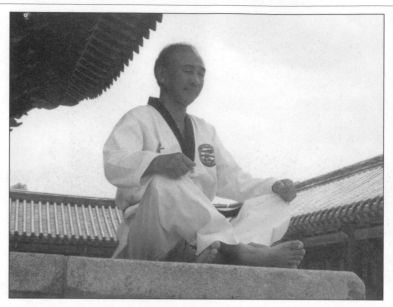

Richard Chun meditating at Bulkook Temple, Kyungju, Korea, 1999.

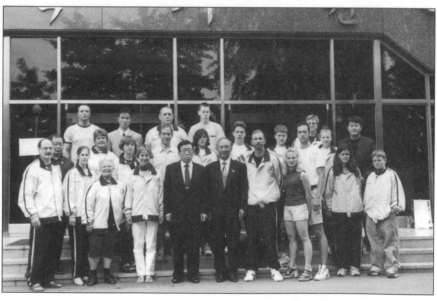

USTA members visiting the Kukkiwon (World Taekwondo Center) in Seoul, Korea. Dr. Un Yong Kim (left), Richard Chun (right), 1999.

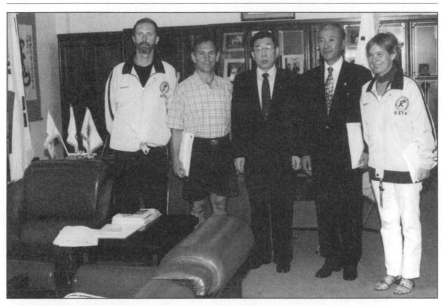

Dr. Un Yong Kim (center), president of the World Taekwondo Federation at his office with Richard Chun and USTA Instructors, 1999.

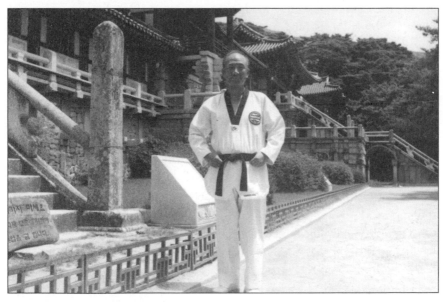

Richard Chun at Bulkook Temple in 1999, where young aristocrats called Hwarangdan trained Taekwondo 2,000 years ago.

ABOUT THE AUTHOR

Richard Chun began studying Taekwondo at the age of 11 under two highly respected teachers in Seoul, Korea: Chong Soo Hong and Ki Whang Kim. He progressed to 9th Dan by Kukkiwon (World Taekwondo Federation) and Moo Duk Kwan after more than fifty years of study, establishing him as one of the highest ranking master instructors in the United States. (9th Dan by Kukkiwon in 1989 and by Moo Duk Kwan in 1981)

A graduate of Yon Sei University in Seoul in 1957, he organized and served as team captain of the Taekwondo Club. Immigrating to the United States in 1962, he earned an M.B.A. in marketing from the School of Business Administration at Long Island University and a Ph.D. in Education. He has been a Professor of Health and Physical Education at Hunter College City University of New York. Dr. Chun has been teaching Taekwondo at his center in New York City for four decades.

He was instrumental in organizing the Annual Universal Taekwondo Championships in the 1960's. He was appointed head coach of the U.S.A. Taekwondo team in 1973 for the first World Taekwondo Championships in Seoul. He has traveled and lectured extensively at local Taekwondo schools around the country as well as made appearances on TV talk shows. He went on to establish the United States Taekwondo Association in 1980 and has served as its President as well as assisted in the organization of Taekwondo as an event in the 1988 Olympics. Dr. Chun has since served as Senior International Referee for championships and the Olympics. In the fall of 1999, Dr. Chun was appointed as a Special Assistant to the President of the World Taekwondo Federation, Dr. Un Yong Kim. He continues to train senior black belts around the world and was inducted into the Black Belt Hall of Fame by *Black Belt* Magazine in 1979.

Taekwondo Spirit and Practice is his fifth book. His other books are Tae Kwon Do and *Advancing in Tae Kwon Do*, both published by Harper-Collins and still in print. *Tae Kwon Do Moo Duk Kwan, Volumes I and II* are published by Ohara Publications. These books are on technique in the art of Taekwondo. He has also produced a number of instructional videos on self-defense.

Dr. Chun has also been a member of the Lions Clubs International for over thirty years, where he has served as District Governor in New York. He is married with two children.

INDEX

BOOKS FROM YMAA PUBLICATION CENTER

YMAA PUBLICATION CENTER 楊氏東方文化出版中心

4354 Washington Street Roslindale, MA 02131

1-800-669-8892 • ymaa@aol.com • www.ymaa.com

VIDEOS FROM YMAA PUBLICATION CENTER

YM
4354
1-80